On Mood Swings

The Psychobiology of Elation and Depression

Dr. Suzanne Shad-Somers
The Psychobiology of Elation & Depression
on Mood Swings

On Mood Swings
The Psychobiology of Elation and Depression

Susanne P. Schad-Somers, Ph.D.

Private Practice
New York, New York
and New School for Social Research
New York, New York

Foreword by
Francis G. Mas, M.D.

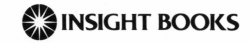 **INSIGHT BOOKS**

Plenum Press • New York and London

Library of Congress Cataloging-in-Publication Data

Schad-Somers, Susanne P. (Susanne Petra), 1939-
   On mood swings : the psychobiology of elation and depression
 Susanne P. Schad-Somers ; foreword by Francis G. Mas.
      p.   cm.
   "Insight books."
   Includes bibliographical references.
   Includes index.
   ISBN 0-306-43562-4
   1. Affective disorders--Physiological aspects. 2. Biological
 psychiatry. I. Title.
   [DNLM: 1. Affective Disorders--psychology. 2. Depression-
 -psychology. WM 171 S292o]
 RC537.S38 1990
 616.85'27--dc20
 DNLM/DLC
 for Library of Congress   90-7672
                                                               CIP

Grateful acknowledgement is made for permission to reprint excerpts from the
following material:

The Little Prince by Antoine de Saint-Exupéry. Copyright 1943 and renewed © 1971
   by Harcourt Brace Jovanovich, Inc. Reprinted by permission.

Diagnostic and Statistical Manual of Mental Disorders, Third Edition, Revised.
© 1987 American Psychiatric Association. Reprinted by permission.

© 1990 Plenum Press, New York
A Division of Plenum Publishing Corporation
233 Spring Street, New York, N.Y. 10013

An Insight Book

Printed in the United States of America

This book is for J.A.S.

Foreword

Fiat Lux. —Genesis 1:1

In earlier times, when life, or rather the perception of life, was simpler, the nature of light was felt to be a God-given "obvious" entity. However, as knowledge evolved, the complicated nature of this phenomenon became more apparent, to such an extent that earlier in this century its complexity appeared to be unfathomable.

Two perfectly valid groups of experiments, giving strikingly opposite results, were then showing light to be "either" a corpuscle "or" a wave, thus creating much confusion. Quantum theory solved this apparent contradiction by devising sets of equations representing light to have the capacity to act both as a wave "and" as a corpuscle. This formulation was a close enough representation of an intrinsic reality to be fully operational and to allow for further major advances in physics.

I believe that studies of the nature of psychopathology and its related therapeutics can benefit from the analysis of such a conceptual evolution. In this book, Dr. Schad-Somers is, in fact, following a similar approach by showing the critical importance of psychosocial *and* biological factors in mental health. Each human being can be seen as a unique blend of these ever-evolving, ever-interacting components which cannot be artificially separated without risks. This notion is equally crucial to people like Dr. Schad-Somers, who is a psychotherapist, and to those who, like myself, work as a neuropsychiatrist called to evaluate and treat the possible biological distortions in a given psychopathological case.

To use a further metaphor, we often find ourselves in the position of someone listening to a musician playing in the next room behind a closed door, analyzing the pitch, clarity, and tempo, as well as the choice of the melody, while at the same time trying to discriminate between playing techniques and instrument-related idiosyncrasies and structural anomalies. This task was at one point practically impossible, but has recently become much easier as a set of basic rules allow for better clinical discrimination and subsequent individualized therapeutic modalities. The barrier of the closed door is also now more permeable as imaging techniques can generate a better visualization of the structure as well as functional integrity of the "hands-instrument complex" (i.e., the brain).

Such a progress may be timely, as, to pursue our analogy, the "musical partition" to be read by mankind may become harder in an ever increasing fashion. Unless "techniques" and "instrumental reliability" keep pace, one may witness large-scale suffering and concomitant further attempts at self-treatment with a variety of "street" drugs. Meanwhile, the basic and clinical neurosciences' exponential growth over the past 40 years has already brought us a large body of knowledge. Sadly, it is most often unused or misused because of an age-old persistently misleading mind-body dichotomy which is often so crystallized as to present an unsurmountable therapeutic challenge.

Therefore, one has to be particularly grateful to Dr. Schad-Somers for presenting the multifactorial reality hiding behind the often deceptive appearances of psychopathology. Her book has the further merit of articulating the psychobiological uniqueness of each individual within a larger sociohistorical and evolutionary context. Such an approach is most welcome, as well as sorely needed, and can best be summarized by quoting T. S. Eliot:

Round and round the circle
Completing the charm
So the knot be unknotted
The cross be uncrossed
The crooked be made straight
And the curse be ended.

Francis G. Mas, M.D.
Department of Psychiatry
New York University Medical School

Acknowledgments

The fact that this manuscript got done on time is only due to the fact that Pamela White Hadas gently but very firmly coerced the author—a dyslexic and a confirmed technophobe—to jump headlong into the twentieth century by getting a computer. Furthermore, and that is the sign of true friendship, she retyped and edited countless manuscript pages which were lost to that voracious electronic beast. Similarly, Jean Mundy, time and again, dropped whatever she was doing, jumped into her car and bailed me out of assorted mechanical jams. She too read and retyped several sections of this book. I am immensely grateful to both of them.

As for Peter from Spread the Word Computer Services in Sag Harbor: Consider it done.

Morris Stein—again—extended himself beyond the call of duty, even friendship, by not only reading and critiquing four exceedingly unkempt chapters, but doing so in the space of a weekend and then leaving five single-spaced pages of comments on my front porch.

I am grateful to Stanley Schachter for roasting me over the coals as unmercifully as he did. As a result I now have a most extensive collection of modifiers, one that undoubtedly (or for the most part, perhaps) will be large enough to last me for the rest of my life.

Regina Cherry, with an unerring nose for split infinitives and missing commas, read each and every page with great care, hunting down non sequiturs and examples of sloppy thinking and accepting no shortcuts. Her labors are profoundly appreciated.

My debt to Francis Mas is twofold; one: as my psychopharmacologist he has always medicated my depressed patients expertly. Moreover, in the face of acute mania he has shown himself to be as unflappable as I am not. Two: as a reader, he devoted an enormous amount of time to the task of editing all those chapters involving biology. Most important, from start to finish he consistently communicated his conviction that the job of writing this book was a necessary and important one.

As always, I believe that the ultimate gratitude belongs to my patients who, after all, taught me at least as much as I taught them. While I learned, threading my way through all sorts of conceptual and factual confusions, they waited patiently, trusting that there would be an adequate degree of understanding in the end. For all those times when I accused some of them of "just acting out" and for those instances when I accepted the explanation of "mood disorder" too readily, I apologize.

Last, and decidedly least, a small measure of thanks goes to Eurydice, a Tibetan terrier whose pawprints, literally and figuratively, are all over these pages, for graciously agreeing to only chase the ticker tape from the computer printout instead of the actual pages.

Susanne P. Schad-Somers

East Hampton, New York

Contents

On Mood Swings

Introduction

As our century draws to a close, many advances have been made in the fields of medicine and psychology. However, with respect to the question, what causes people to become depressed, we still have at least four competing schools of thought. The remedies advocated vary accordingly.

Biopsychiatry claims that depression essentially reflects some biochemical disturbance in the brain. Andreason (1982), one of the leading proponents of this approach, concedes that sometimes episodes of illness are triggered by unfortunate life events; but she goes on to say the basic causes lie in the biology of what she calls *The Broken Brain*. Consequently, the best way to treat these abnormalities in brain function is through somatic therapies.

Cognitive therapists, on the other hand, argue that depression is due to some distortion in thinking. Depressed people tend to concentrate on the worst aspects of themselves, their world, their circumstances, and their future. Their software is skewed in the direction of pessimism and self-blame. Treatment, which for some practitioners includes hypnosis, involves restructuring the patients' "faulty" thinking and perceiving, and showing them how to make a more accurate assessment of their lives.

Psychoanalysis focuses on childhood events, fantasies, and feelings, and their respective impact on the vicissitudes of the instincts, namely libido and aggression and, correspondingly, the complex defensive structures that were erected to deal with all the possible conflicts to which they can give rise. The recovery of events and the feelings and fantasies connected with them is the cure.

Sociologists explain depression as the result of miserable lives, poverty, prejudice, social isolation, being trapped in dead-end jobs or marriages, etc.—in other words, the reality of people's circumstances is the basic problem. Furthermore, they point out, a society which raises expectations with respect to the possibilities for success, social mobility, and financial security, without providing the avenues to obtain these goals, puts people at risk for depression because if they do not succeed, they believe that they have no one but themselves to blame for their failure. Furthermore, to the extent that traditional institutions, such as family and the church, have lost their importance as buffers against feelings of helplessness and hopelessness, with no alternatives to replace them, coping with individual "failure" may feel like clearing an insurmountable hurdle.

For people who are experiencing a debilitating depression, this state of affairs, i.e., the variety of conceptual and practical approaches, is no joking matter if they desire to feel better and, therefore, have to decide who to ask for help or, alternatively, who to blame if the therapy chosen fails to work. Wrong doctor or wrong medicine?

Not all the data are in yet to answer the question of what causes depression. However, if we cannot yet answer many questions pertaining to the multiple causes of depression, biochemistry and neuroscience have vastly advanced our understanding of that phenomenon. In fact, this development may be occurring at a speed in excess of what our collective consciousness may be ready to absorb all at once. This intellectual development has recently prompted Eric Kandel (1989) to comment

> when social historians look upon the second half of the 20th century, they are likely to acknowledge that the most interesting insights into our understanding of the mind will not have come from

the traditional disciplines concerned with the mind; they will not
have come from philosophy or from the arts, nor from psychoanalysis or even from cognitive psychology, but from biology, and
specifically from molecular biology and from neurobiology. (p. 103)

While biology alone cannot unlock the mysteries of mind,
mood, and motivation, the field loosely called psychobiology
does a pretty good job in showing us where to look in the so-
called nature-nurture dilemma. To be specific:

Historically, thanks in no small measure to the experimental
trials and tribulations of a lowly sea snail, the *Aplysia Californica*,
psychotherapy, or the talking cure, is beginning to acquire a
sound theoretical base and the potential for markedly increased
effectiveness in ways it never could have done before.

In addition, the veritable avalanche of findings in the fields
of psychobiology, genetics, psychopharmacology, brain research, ethology, etc., has resulted in two major advances in the
treatment of mental illness.

One: We are now beginning to understand why it is that
specific interactions, particularly those between parents and
children or therapists and patients, such as talking or stroking,
scolding or battering, can result in long-lasting changes in the
neural machinery of the people so involved. This may not sound
very revolutionary; after all, it is something that every parent
"knows" instinctively. Soothing talk and the laying on of hands
has been part of the therapeutic armamentarium of healers since
the time of the cave. What has changed is the nature of our
knowledge, how we know what we "know." When we therapists talk with our patients today, our justification for doing so is
no longer because Sigmund Freud said it works, but because we
are beginning to understand biologically how mental processes
and interactions can affect the brain and the central nervous
system and how, at least to some extent, we are beginning to
measure these changes empirically (John, Prichep, Friedman, &
Easton, 1988).

Freud, in his 1895 "Project for a Scientific Psychology," had
hoped that one day we would be able to map the neurological

substratum of our mental life, and in some of his hunches on how this works he was instinctively right; for example, he postulated that pleasure pathways are established through learning. But in some other guesses of his he was not so fortunate, because the life sciences and, in particular, the neurology of his time could not yet supply him with the necessary information to complete the "Project." Sadly, but accurately, he had to conclude that

> we know two kinds of things about what we call our psyche (or mental life): firstly, its bodily organ and scene of action, the brain (or nervous system) and, on the other hand, our acts of consciousness, which are immediate data and cannot be further explained by any sort of description. Everything that lies in between is unknown to us, and the data do not include any direct relation between those two terminal points of our knowledge. (1949, p.1)

As a consequence, until one or two decades ago, the only way we could communicate with each other, with our patients, and with the public at large was through metaphors or analogies; in other words, constructs that have no real counterpart in the brain or the central nervous system. In the absence of biological information, and because we have to call mental processes and phenomena something, we did our work as if our metaphors for the various components of our mental life were real entities. For example, people obviously differ in their ability and determination to get to where they are going and to successfully navigate their way through the demands of what we call the reality principle. We refer to that entity as ego strength and, as metaphors go, it has served us pretty well in doing our work in spite of the fact that there is nothing in our brains that can be identified as an ego. It designates a composite of a variety of psychological and cognitive phenomena, comparable to an index of air quality.

Before the workings of the brain and central nervous system were better understood, the mapping out of our psyche was a hit-or-miss affair, guided for the most part by Freud's genius, the principle of good fit and, sometimes, the fancy of the ambitious and imaginative. Some concepts proved to be enduring, while others made a splash for a short while and then went the way of all fads. Orgone boxes are mostly museum pieces and the notion of a death instinct is rapidly losing adherents. Given what we have learned about the biological substratum of the mind and the different feedback loops between different systems and organs, and between the mind and the brain, we are slowly approaching the point where we are able to sort through the various theories and the corresponding metaphors that have accumulated in the last hundred years and to sort out the possible from the impossible, the probable from the improbable, and to bring some of our theories into line with the advances made in the biological sciences, even if that means kicking an occasional sacred cow.

What are some of the things we are learning from biology? In a singularly elegant and deceptively simple experiment conducted by Eric R. Kandel, biologists were able to demonstrate for the first time, and conclusively, that cells—at least in the case of the sea snail—will learn from experience. In testing such a daring hypothesis clearly and unambiguously, scientists wanted an organism as uncomplicated as possible in its physiological structure and one which can be easily observed. The *Aplysia* was a perfect candidate. If its syphon or spout is tapped, this snail will withdraw its gills. This is a reflex, a part of the genetic makeup of this particular animal. But instead of this reflex being immutable, the researchers found that if they continuously tapped the spout, the snail stopped responding. This lack of reaction is not because the snail got tired or bored, but because the repetitive touch alters the neurons in the snail's gill-withdrawing circuit in such a way that the message system connecting the outside of the head with the inside slowly changes. In other words, the organism of the snail adapts to noxious and continuous stimuli with long-lasting cellular changes which can be studied in detail.

While it will be some time before we can duplicate these findings in organisms as complex as human beings, the basic principle, namely that cells can remember, that they are not biological givens, but dynamic parts of a functional network, applies to snails and man alike. Meanwhile, through innumerable experiments with different animals, and through the observations of psychologically deprived children, we are learning a great deal about how different psychological and social experiences shape the organism—its soma the "megasystem"—with behavioral results ranging from the most benign to the truly catastrophic.

In a fatal experiment—fatal for the subjects, that is—having to do with the origins of language, Frederick Barbarossa demonstrated a long time ago that infants whose physiological needs are met, but who receive no further care such as being held, spoken to, rocked, etc., will in fact die within their first year of life. In our time, Harry F. Harlow and his colleagues have shown that socially and psychologically deprived monkey babies will grow into adults incapable of such elementary tasks as mating or raising their young. Findings such as those have made it necessary to redefine the concept of "instinct" as a built-in biological push-button system. There is now enough evidence to support the view that all animals—man included—are born with a genetically determined blueprint for a vast array of behavioral systems, such as procreation, food acquisition, and sociability; but it requires continuous and nontraumatic social interactions with a primary caretaker and with peers for these systems to unfold. These systems, given a traumatic environment, can be retarded in their development; but they can also be rehabilitated through methods not too dissimilar from those through which they would have developed in a more benign environment.

As anybody knows who has ever taken in an abused or abandoned pup, the process of reestablishing trust and consequent physical and emotional health follows very predictable and predetermined steps, allowing for no shortcuts. Until the reflex that is based on the equation "human hand equals punishment" is extinguished, the pup cannot store memories of gratifying interactions with a human. Similarly, when a patient, after years of plunging into a profound depression every time the therapist leaves for vacation, is finally able to maintain a steady sense of connectedness and an absence of that immobilizing despondency, that patient has acquired what we call "object constancy," the emotional and cognitive ability to visualize and to feel the object or person even if he or she is physically absent. As a consequence, the mind does not signal "depressive reaction" to the central nervous system and the patient remains calm and contented, knowing the object is safe and bound to return. In our clinical lingo we say that the soothing aspects of the interaction with the therapist have been "internalized" to such an extent that it affects the total organism. Put differently, the evidence is mounting that the stuff that happens on the couch on a weekly basis—the talking cure—if it is successful—will bring about changes in the neural machinery of the brain. We never knew that before; we only saw behavioral changes without knowing how they came about. However, winning the trust of an abandoned pup and dealing with an abandonment depression in an adult human are not the same thing.

What complicates matters in humans immensely is the fact we have minds that can be tricky indeed, ingenious enough to exalt a state of clinical depression, homicidal rage, mania or obsession to the status of a religion or political dogma and thus not subject to any therapeutic intervention.

The attempts at understanding the unhappy outcomes of unfortunate childhoods prompted Freud to postulate such biologically untenable forces as a death instinct, defined as the desire of all organisms to return to an inorganic state. While we are still far from having at our disposal a psychobiology of self-destruction, we do know that masochism, for example, is not the manifestation of an instinct or drive, but a learned behavior—soft-wired into the psyche, the brain and the central nervous system—and quite accessible to psychotherapeutic intervention. In a similar vein, when we look at an adolescent suicide or a midlife depression, we can surmise quite a bit about the corresponding or underlying biological, i.e., neurohormonal, processes in the brain. Complementing this, we do have a growing arsenal of psychoanalytic constructs that are not only consonant with the relevant biology, but also look and treat such depressions as the outcome of a life-long interaction between psychological, social, and biological forces.

One of the most intuitive psychoanalysts, Michael Balint (1968), coined the term "basic fault," an analogy borrowed from geology. It designates a profound vulnerability in the psyche of some people which resembles the St. Andreas fault in California. For most of the time, all goes well. But given specific acute or chronic stresses on the fault lines, major upheavals will result. This is not only a very useful and poetic concept but one for which the brain researchers are beginning to find supportive evidence. Like its geological counterpart, it is not a single entity, but consists of a number of interrelated factors, such as genetic vulnerabilities, coupled with specific childhood traumas which, in conjunction with acute stresses in adult life, will quite predictably trigger an emotional earthquake.

When the friends of an adolescent suicide recall only "such a happy child," they may be quite right. What they saw was a seemingly untroubled youngster; what they could not or would not see were the underlying fault lines. Given a particularly protective environment, such as a remote farm or a monastery, people with such fault lines may well go through life without any major eruptions. Unfortunately, such safe niches are rare in modern industrialized society. Along similar lines, the analyst Masud Khan (1974) speaks about the "protective shield," the infant's (and later the adult's) ability to screen out noxious noises and other stimuli that impinge on the organism. This "shield" is what allows the infant to tolerate noise and to sleep peacefully in even a crowded subway car. The protective shield is thought to be acquired in response to empathic mothering; it is as if the infant were literally capable of soaking up the soothing and comforting presence of the caretaker, mother or father. Manic patients and some depressives are notoriously deficient in this regard; overstimulation is a constant complaint. The biological correlate of the protective shield, i.e., what happens in the brain, appears to be the maturation of the central nervous system, the laying down of those neural connections that the organism can employ to protect itself from overstimulation and trauma. The late analyst Heinz Kohut (1971) gave that process the somewhat inelegant term "transmuting internalizations" and, more than most analysts, he stressed the fact that our ability for mood regulation and self-soothing is acquired in early infancy in response to the empathy of the primary caretaker. Parents who, for whatever reasons, fail their offspring in this process may raise children who are somewhat handicapped in their ability to withstand overstimulation, and to weather disappointments, such as abandonments and personal or vocational failures. If, in addition, these children have inherited a genetic vulnerability towards affective disorders, i.e., unipolar or bipolar depression or schizophrenia, they are at serious risk for these disorders.

On the whole, what biology is teaching us is that in understanding the human psyche we come closer to the truth if we use concepts such as "behavioral systems" instead of "drives," "attachment behavior" instead of "libido," and "arousal" instead of "discharge." Equally important is the fact that we now have solid reasons to believe that the much misused and maligned term "corrective parenting," to describe the process of psychotherapy, has a sound basis in reality. Adult cells, too, are dynamic entities and consequently they too can remember. They can learn as well as unlearn. The human mind, with all its complexity and power, can be used in many therapeutic modalities to accomplish many positive changes.

The second major advance in our field is a much better understanding of the ways in which moods or affects are reflected in or caused by the electrochemical transmission system in our central nervous system and in our brain. As a result, we now have the possibility of using drug therapy with those patients for whom the talking cure is necessary but not sufficient, i.e., the various subtypes of schizophrenia, people suffering from mania or clinical depression, obsessive-compulsive disorders, some anxiety disorders, and phobics. After all, emotions do not take place in a physical vacuum, they are biological events that can involve the entire organism, ranging from total immobilization to near-fatal feats of endurance and subsequent exhaustion.

The depressed person is depressed not just mentally but also physiologically, a phenomenon that we call "psychomotor retardation." The person experiencing this type of clinical depression feels as if he or she had glue in their arteries instead of blood, the entire body is shut down, particularly the brain and the central nervous system. The tendency of organisms to respond with depression exists in many of the more evolved species because, strange as this may sound, it is adaptive and has an evolutionary advantage. The baby animal who gets separated from the group should shut down, since persistent distress signals would attract predators, and excessive movement would use up precious reserves of energy. What we call an abandonment depression in humans is in animal cubs or pups or chicks the only intelligent response to being lost in the wild. For the next couple of million years we are probably stuck with that evolutionary inheritance.

Manic, or rather manic-depressive patients (bipolar depression) find themselves on an unstoppable emotional roller coaster. During the manic phase the organism goes into "overdrive," with thoughts, feelings, and movements going at 200 miles per hour. A person in the throes of an acute mood disorder thinks and acts in ways that are congruent with that particular disorder, including the feeling that the mood or affect is out of control. For example, the lover, depressed and with a broken heart, will argue convincingly that there is no chance on earth of ever finding another human worthy of love, that all hope of ever feeling happy again is absurd and that he or she is so unworthy that suicide would be the best solution, not only for the abandoned lover, but also for the world as a whole; that the lover and the whole world should not have to put up with such a miserable wretch. Similarly, the manic-depressive, during the manic phase, will find it perfectly normal to spend more money in an hour than he will earn in a lifetime, and he will try to convince others to invest in that same wonderful opportunity for un- limited wealth. Quite a few manic suicides have been due to the fact that the patient truly thought he or she could fly or cross an interstate highway in less than 60 seconds. In other words, ma- nia and depression can seriously impair a person's cognitive functioning, i.e., his ability to respond appropriately to clear and present dangers and his awareness of physical and mental limitations.

We know that the brain chemistry of patients in these states is clearly disturbed. One or several of the neurotransmitters, the chemicals responsible for carrying messages from one nerve cell to another do so in greater or lesser volume or quantity, and/or they are metabolized abnormally. The electrical activity in the brain of the mood-disordered person differs significantly from that of normal controls. These abnormalities can be measured: hormonal challenger tests, PET scans, EEG, etc. As for deter- mining the type and the seriousness of a disorder, the activity of the different neurotransmitters across the synapse between nerve cells is the manifestation of the mood disorder most acces- sible to us. We have come a long way in understanding and measuring it, and psychopharmacologists are finding more and more effective ways of influencing neurotransmitter activity and corresponding mood disorders with the help of drugs. That, however, does not necessarily mean that the business in the synapse is the ultimate cause of the mood disorder. Rather, this is the point of entry, as it were, the stuff we can do something about. The gridlock on Fifth Avenue may have as its ultimate cause a stalled subway car in Brooklyn; but as long as we can double the traffic lanes going out of Manhattan, the jam on Fifth Avenue may be sufficiently alleviated. Properly administered drugs will, more often than not, restore a depressed person to normal functioning. The same can happen in response to thera- peutic or psychosocial interventions. A faithless lover returned to his beloved is the greatest antidepressant of all. In fact, a very elegant and controlled study of depressed women in an outpatient clinic in London clearly demonstrated that on the average what is called "social skills training" was slightly more effective in treating mild or moderate depression than the administration of antidepressant drugs. On the other hand, psychotherapy alone with severe depressives and many manic-depressives can be a very dangerous waste of time and may easily have a fatal outcome. A patient, full of insight, may kill himself.

Some of the more skillful and intuitive psychoanalysts of the past, Edith Jacobson (1971) for one, always felt that bipolar disorders are not caused by psychological factors alone, and they suspected some unknown but probably inborn constitutional factors. We now know what some of these are. First and foremost, the vulnerability towards mood disorders is inherited. Secondly, specific physiological factors such as changes in the hormonal balance and certain drugs, be they therapeutic or recreational, can trigger an affective disorder in vulnerable individuals. However, genetic vulnerability or predisposition is only part of the story. The environment determines whether or not an affective disorder will in fact develop, and it will also influence its severity. Both unipolar and bipolar depressions, as well as alcoholism, tend to run in families, but they do so for at least two reasons. A mood-disordered parent, grandparent, or sibling is likely to significantly disturb the family equilibrium, and many mood disorders are covered over by alcoholism. Consequently, the children of such families are very often doubly handicapped: having to deal with a genetic predisposition and a less than optimal and sometimes disastrous environment. A mood-disordered alcoholic parent can make life a living hell for a child; it may even destroy the more vulnerable among them.

Psychotherapy is still an art, the art of sensing with any given patient what the specific configuration of the disorder might be and how to maximize the effectiveness of the different treatment modalities or approaches. Psychopharmacology, besides forcing us to think more clearly, has made us much more effective with some patients; it is quite literally saving the lives of some others.

Why some psychoanalysts and psychotherapists still look at the use of drugs as an undesirable shortcut, an attempt to eliminate the process of "working it through," is largely incomprehensible, for two reasons: In the course of "working it through," a patient may lose years of what could be a productive life, years that can never be regained; he may wreck important professional and educational chances that may never be offered again, and, what is worse, the patient may never work it through because the unruly brain chemistry cannot be brought to heel. One can have patients dripping with insights, knowing all the right things to do to change their lives for the better, but who are too depressed or too manic to implement their good intentions. Conversely, the depressed person who is medicated is not cured; only medicated. Lifelong habits, unconscious hidden agendas, unresolved conflicts, and all the other aspects of a depressed and depressing life-style are still present and have to be addressed and worked through as they do with every other patient. After all, affective disorder is rarely a sufficient diagnosis, since it can occur along the entire continuum of ego impairment, from neurotic to character disorder to borderline structure to psychotic. Furthermore, within each of these categories people can be masochistic, paranoid, obsessional, or can exhibit any other interpersonal or intrapsychic orientation. To deal with those problems is the psychotherapeutic task, while the drug treatment provides the internal climate within which these changes become possible.

In other words, a mood disorder is a complex psychobiological event, the culmination of various processes into "a final common pathway" (Akiskal & McKinney, 1973). The elements contributing to it are the following: (1) Genetic vulnerability; (2) developmental events, such as early object loss, which leave the organism vulnerable to similar events in adult life, such as divorce, loss of a spouse, etc.; (3) chronic or acute stresses that overwhelm the coping mechanism of the organism;

(4) physiological stressors such as certain viral infections, child-birth, hypothyroidism, etc.; (5) personality traits, such as shyness or introversion which predispose an individual towards social isolation; and (6) variables that belong to a different sphere but can act as important moderators, namely psycho-pathology, not necessarily related to mood disorders, as, for example sociopathy, which means that a depressed crook on medication is still a crook and will find ways around the depression or its effects. He may be too depressed to write his term papers, but he will know where to buy, plagiarize, or to steal them.

The structure of this book is based on the principal questions raised here. To begin with, the life histories of a handful of people have been chosen to illustrate the diversity of the phenomenon called depression. They include unipolar (depression) and bipolar (manic-depressive) depression—some of these people sought treatment and others did not; and the tragic case of one patient who consistently got the wrong kind of help. A brief overview of the history of Western society's understanding of mental illness in general and mood disorders in particular should explain why the Western life sciences had so many difficulties in conceiving of the dialectic underlying the concept of "psychobiology." Two separate chapters will examine homo sapiens as a primarily symbolic animal (psyche) and another, in contrast, examines the purely physiological machinery, i.e., cell communication and neurochemistry. Chapter six merely attempts to convey some of the flavor of the excitement generated by psychobiology, presenting just a few of the findings fairly unsystematically, and in spite of the fact that some of them are still considered to be somewhat controversial. Before we can look at how depression might best be treated, we need to know how mood regulation is acquired in early childhood, what typically goes wrong in the early lives of people who become depressed and, specifically, how this applies to the patients presented in the first and second chapters. Chapter seven examines these questions. Chapter eight then attempts to connect some of the findings from biology to the working of the "talking cure," while Chapter nine focuses on the treatment problems that are specific for people who suffer from depression and who are also treated with drugs, the three S's, namely shame, stigma, and suicide. Finally, in Chapter ten we will return to our case history material once more in order to see what and how psycho-therapy, life, medical care, or drug treatment actually affected the lives of those people.

While it is still true that both mania and depression can be potentially life-threatening disorders, we have never been in a better position to deal with them as we are now. And if in addition to the advances made by biology and its related sci-ences we can tap some of the innovations made by the new field of behavioral medicine and apply them to regulate dysfunctions of the brain and the central nervous system, the future looks brighter yet.

CHAPTER ONE

Jack

The Wrong Kind of Help

In the summer of 1965, for the first time in almost 20 years, Jack had solid reasons to believe that his long struggle with mental illness was finally won. One evening, he and his wife-to-be were discussing the guest list for their upcoming wedding, when a phone call from Jack's son brought disturbing news: Jack's former sister-in-law and Jack's best friend had both been arrested at a civil rights demonstration and were, at that moment, in jail. This phone call set a process in motion that has continued to this day. During that particular time in his life, Jack had all the evidence that he was intact as a person, that he lived life as he had always wanted to, and his hopes for the future were quite justified. This had not come about easily.

When Jack was 18, and a sophomore at Columbia University, his life had suddenly spun out of control. He had been very politically active as a student, involved in Marxist causes, protesting his narrow bourgeois Catholic background, and he had become the proverbial angry young man—angry and intense, too intense. In the course of one particularly powerful fit of anger and depression Jack tried to drown himself in the bathtub. His mother called the parish priest. He in turn called the police and an ambulance, which took Jack to Bellevue Hospital. This institution, at that time, was rightly known as "the snakepit."

Besides suffering from a case of near-fatal dehydration, Jack was diagnosed as suffering from schizophrenia. He was put into a straitjacket, injected with a massive dose of Thorazine, a powerful psychoactive drug, and with eight attendants holding down this athlete, who stood 6'4" in his stocking feet, he was given a series of 26 electroshocks without benefit of anesthesia. After three months of hospitalization he was discharged. He moved to a small town in another state, became a factory worker, union organizer, and eventually a part-time college student. He married, and a year later he had a son. However, increasingly, Jack felt that he had to move awfully fast in order to accomplish all the goals he had set for himself, and, at the same time, to also provide for his new family. At the age of 28 he became increasingly tense, angry at his wife and fellow workers, his bosses, slept less and less, and suffered increasingly from bouts of depression. Finally he became overtly psychotic. Once he was hospitalized, the original diagnosis—schizophrenia—was amended to "paranoid schizophrenia," due to the fact that he exhibited an "inappropriate distrust of psychiatry and mental hospitals." Jack later used to quip: Even paranoids have real enemies.

In the course of his breakdown, too many ugly things had been said and done for that marriage to survive. The couple divorced. After his discharge from the hospital, Jack returned to work and to school and began a psychoanalytically oriented psychotherapy. To his utter delight, his academic work in college was recognized as being of such quality that it earned him a Woodrow Wilson scholarship for Harvard Graduate School. After a year at Harvard, he transferred his studies to New York, where he met his future wife. He lived on a NIMH grant and held a part-time college teaching position. He was in the process of writing his Master's thesis when he received that fateful phone call. He was 37 years old.

In the course of the last two years, Gerda, his New York

psychiatrist, had helped him in twice-weekly sessions to sort through his conflictual attachments to his family. She was impressed with the progress he had made on that score, and she was delighted when he decided to get married again. Jack had felt that it was vitally important that his bride know his entire life history, including those two breakdowns. Gerda disagreed strongly for several reasons. One, she felt that it was highly unlikely that Jack would ever have another breakdown; two, that it would needlessly frighten his wife and that it would label or stigmatize him in her eyes. Gerda argued that the young woman would suddenly see the diagnosis "schizophrenia" instead of the person. With Gerda's vote of confidence in his mental health, Jack kept the secret to himself. Then, when the phone call came, Jack experienced not even a moment's hesitation in deciding to drop everything he was doing and to drive back to that city where he had lived and worked—and where he had his second breakdown.

Eight hours after he left New York, Jack too was in jail. When his fiancee arrived the following day with an attorney and with bail money, she found a man she had never seen before. The look in his eyes indicated flashes of madness. It bespoke a terrifying night in jail, with brutal beatings and bloody exchanges between the state troopers and the mostly black demonstrators. During the next three days, Jack did what he could, trying to round up white middle-class support and to arrange for inexpensive legal defense for himself as well as for the other demonstrators. The protesters were charged with the usual set of trumped-up charges and a trial date was set for the day after Jack's planned wedding.

Back in New York, life seemingly returned to normal. However, there also was an almost entirely unnoticeable difference. Jack's heart was elsewhere. Though outwardly nothing had changed, Jack's deepest allegiance shifted a little, from his personal life to that entity which then was called "the Movement," and which increasingly rocked all American college campuses. Jack's Master's thesis got postponed; he was too busy attending meetings and political rallies. In the midst of all this hectic activity, Jack stayed up one night with friends. They had all been smoking marijuana, which made his wife sleepy, while it stimulated Jack. While she went to sleep, he grew increasingly agitated.

At six o'clock the following morning he woke her up, requesting quite calmly but unequivocally that she drive him to his psychiatrist, who lived in a suburb. By the time they arrived at Gerda's office, Jack had begun to hallucinate. After speaking to Jack for some time, Gerda decided that the couple should drive home, on their way filling a prescription for Thorazine and for the antidepressant Elavil. They were told to go home just long enough to pack their bags, and then proceed to the country cottage of Jack's brother, until such time when Jack was calmer.

This prescription worked for a while. Nobody knew anything; Jack's wife, a colleague, simply took over his teaching position, and after a few months the couple returned to New York. Though Jack was indeed quite calm, for the next year he was also profoundly depressed. He attended his psychotherapy session regularly and he took his medications faithfully.

However, the only antidepressant that *really* worked for Jack was political activity. Attending intense meetings lifted his spirits though they also caused tension and insomnia. Jack was a very popular and charismatic teacher and his students interpreted his mood swings as signs of dedication to the "the struggle," rather than as an increasing addiction to an activity and a climate that did in fact function as a mood elevator. Though nobody around Jack ever questioned the diagnosis given him, and consequently the treatment prescribed, his wife at times wondered to herself whether there might be such an entity as manic-depressive schizophrenia. Because, what was so striking in his clinical picture, was the enormous contrast between his depressed, remorseful, and extremely insightful moods that prevailed at night, and the self that awoke the following dawn with the overwhelming urge to save the world with yet another sit-in.

After a few years of continuous battle trying to maintain some equilibrium, Jack broke down again, and lost contact with reality. He disappeared, leaving a note that said that "the Cause" made it imperative that he, Jack, move to Harlem. After 72 hours of frantic search, he was found, and returned to the place he feared most in the world—Bellevue Hospital. Eventually he was transferred to Mt. Sinai. Diagnosis and treatment were the same as always. Only, this time, the patient refused to get better. After three months at Mt. Sinai, he left the hospital A.M.A. (against medical advice) and returned home. Too restless to settle in, he soon left his wife and, after a few years, moved to the West Coast.

It seems not too farfetched to assume that his various psychiatrists consoled themselves with the "established fact" that paranoid schizophrenics, besides being extremely uncooperative, are also typically incurable. By that time Jack was 45 years of age, and had become a chronic "schizophrenic," a revolving-door patient, a human being whom just about everybody had given up on. After all, he had been given every combination of drugs imaginable, electroshock treatment, in addition to psychotherapy, and yet he had gotten progressively worse. Now he was a homeless person, disheveled, wandering the streets, provoking or getting into fights, hallucinating, still organizing the masses, with not even the shadow of his former self left. His present whereabouts are unknown.

This represents a not-so-uncommon American psychiatric tragedy. Melvin Konner (1987) has estimated that during the 1960s and 70s, in this country, as many as one-third of patients with manic-depressive (bipolar) disorder were diagnosed as schizophrenics. Though Jack exhibited all the classical symptoms of acute, untreated mania, and even though, between episodes, he went into complete remissions, each of a 10-year duration, a fact which distinguishes the two syndromes, the label schizophrenia was the one that "stuck." That misdiagnosis had two fateful consequences. One, *the single most effective* drug for the treatment of manic-depressive disorder, namely Lithium, was not tried, even once. It was never seriously considered by any of the countless psychiatrists treating him. Two, certain antidepressant drugs, Elavil being one of them, if given to a bipolar patient (manic-depressive) can induce a manic episode, or intensify an existing one.

An alternative interpretation of the "lack of cooperation" on Jack's part could then be that it was part of an heroic effort to remain sane and yet be compliant. His frantic involvement with "the Cause," was, among other things, also a form of self-medication to deal with his deep depressions. The drawback of such intense activity on his part was that it then also quickly ushered in the switch to mania and, with it, eventually, psychosis. His family was forever furious with him because his rational understanding of the detrimental effects of "Movement" meetings on his sanity never lasted very long. Once he became remotely involved he would then pursue the issue with an all-consuming passion that seemed perverse. It never occurred to anybody in his environment that he might have had a good reason for doing what he was trying to do, and that in addition to all the negative reactions that were forthcoming, that he might also deserve a medal for all the demonstrations he chose not to attend.

Jack has been beyond effective help for many years due to the cumulative effect of his bipolar episodes and the corresponding physical and chemical assaults on his brain and his central nervous system. To speculate what his life might have been, given a different diagnosis and, correspondingly, treatment, is too painful to even contemplate.

CHAPTER TWO

Portraits

How the Diagnosis of Depression Is Made

The novelist William Styron (1988) wrote of his own experience with depression:

> What had begun that summer as an off-and-on malaise and vague, spooky restlessness had gained gradual momentum until my nights were without sleep and my days were pervaded by a gray drizzle of unrelenting horror. This horror is virtually indescribable since it bears no relation to normal experience. In depression, a kind of biomedical meltdown, it is the brain as well as the mind that becomes ill—as ill as any other besieged organ. The sick brain plays evil tricks on its inhabiting spirit. Slowly overwhelmed by the struggle, the intellect blurs into stupidity. All capacity for pleasure disappears, and despair maintains a merciless daily drumming. The smallest commonplace of domestic life, so amiable to the healthy mind, lacerates like a blade.

Fearing suicide and not trusting either psychotherapy or anti-depressant drugs to adequately protect him from self-destruction, Styron hospitalized himself until the suicidal danger had passed, and the depression had lifted of its own accord. Styron wrote the essay from which I just quoted, in response to the many literary inquiries into Primo Levi's so-called "failure of nerve" that was assumed to have precipitated Levi's suicide.

What Styron, rightly, wants us to appreciate is the fact that a clinical depression can be an entirely autonomous event.

When we say that a person is depressed, we are referring to a wide spectrum of subjective experiences and objective symptoms. At one end of the spectrum there is the down mood that everybody occasionally experiences, the passing blues following life's predictable or not-so-predictable disappointments and losses; and at the other end there is the experience of a living hell, one which the victims feel they cannot and will not endure beyond a certain point. In those instances suicide is but one solution.

A classificatory scheme of, for example, respiratory disorders is a fairly objective and uniform affair. We know more or less the different causal factors, sites and modes of action, symptom clusters, and therefore the types and the range of possible treatments. For the diagnosis and treatment of depression we have no such thing. In fact we don't even know how many different syndromes might be subsumed under the same term. What we do have are some hard facts, a mélange of more or less plausible hypotheses, with varying amounts of empirical evidence to support them, many divergent theories, and countless opinions. Any diagnostic schema, today, has to incorporate these various elements in terms of congruence, viability, and, ultimately, best fit. While there is no *one* theory of what causes depression, we nevertheless have come a long way in being able at least to discard some of the more baroque claims about causality and classification such as "damned-up sexual energy," or the "death instinct directed at the self." In separating those propositions that are empirically probable from those that seem highly improbable in light of current biological knowledge, we are now in a much better position to give at least an overview of the different types of depression and to offer some psychobiological explanations for their causes. While those explanations are still often tentative, and far from complete, they do nevertheless give us some very effective tools with which treat a respectable percentage of depressed people in such a way that both the patient and the therapist agree that the condition has clearly improved. Before we get into the clinical details of what causes depression, which will be done in Chapter Seven, it seems useful first to give an overview of all the established symptoms of mood disorders.

Clinically, a depression is much more than merely a depressed mood. It is a syndrome involving some or all of the following dimensions which, briefly and schematically summarized, can involve the following: (1) Mood: people can be down or they can be elated, irritable, hostile, chronically enraged, tearful, or on top of the world; (2) cognition: affective disorders can affect memory, selective attention and retrieval, processing of information, concentration and reality-testing; (3) motivation: the normal motivational matrix of pleasure and pain, reward and punishment, approach and avoidance is disrupted; (4) attitudes: the perception of self changes, either in the direction of helplessness, hopelessness, vulnerability, dependency, and incompetence, or its manic obverse, namely omnipotence and grandiosity. The vision of gloom and doom of the depressive has as its mirror an image of invincibility and elation of the manic patient; and (5) somatic: i.e., psychomotor and vegetative functions: psychomotor agitation or psychomotor retardation, sleep disturbances, loss of general interest, increased or decreased food consumption, sex drive, and abnormal digestive processes are all typical symptoms of a more severe depression. Depressions can be mild or severe and they range from a single episode to recurrent or chronic conditions.

During the 1970s, the chaotic state of diagnostic affairs with respect to almost all psychiatric disorders motivated the American Psychiatric Association to compile a definitive diagnostic manual so that, if nothing else, psychiatrists would use a uniform set of terms when speaking about similar or identical psychiatric pictures. Without laying claims to causality, they classified psychiatric syndromes according to the frequencies with which they appeared in specific groups of patients. The classificatory principle is descriptive, or phenomenological, i.e., counting and describing in terms of observable symptoms, rather than etiological, i.e., attempting to categorize on the basis of causality. The result is known as DSM–III—*Diagnostic and Statistical Manual of Mental Disorders*—(APA 1980).

For a patient's experience to qualify as a major depressive episode the following criteria have to be met:

> The essential feature is either a dysphoric mood, or loss of interest or pleasure in all or almost all usual activities or pastimes. The disturbance is prominent, relatively persistent, and associated with other symptoms of the depressive syndrome. These symptoms include appetite disturbance, changes in weight, sleep disturbance, psychomotor agitation or retardation, decreased energy, feelings of worthlessness or guilt, difficulty concentrating or thinking, and thoughts of death or suicide or suicidal attempts.
>
> An individual with a depressive syndrome will usually describe his or her mood as depressed, sad, hopeless, discouraged, down in the dumps, or in terms of some other colloquial variant. Sometimes, however, the mood disturbance may not be expressed as a synonym for depressive mood, but rather as a complaint of 'not caring anymore,' or as a painful inability to experience pleasure.
>
> Loss of interest or pleasure is probably always present in a major depressive episode to some degree, but the individual may not complain of this or even be aware of the loss, although family members may notice it. Withdrawal from friends and family and neglect of avocations that were previously of pleasure are common.
>
> Psychomotor agitation takes the form of inability to sit still, pacing, hand-wringing, pulling or rubbing of hair, skin, clothing, or other objects, outbursts of complaining or shouting, or pressure of speech. Psychomotor retardation may take the form of slowed speech, increased pauses before answering, low or monotonous speech, slowed body movements, a markedly decreased amount of speech (poverty of speech) or muteness. A decrease in energy level is almost invariably present, and is experienced as sustained fatigue even in the absence of physical exertion. The smallest task may seem difficult or impossible to accomplish.
>
> Difficulty in concentrating, slowed thinking, and indecisiveness are frequent. The individual may complain of memory difficulty and appear easily distracted.

> The sense of worthlessness varies from feelings of inadequacy to completely unrealistic negative evaluations of one's worth. The individual may reproach himself or herself for minor failings that are exaggerated and search the environment for clues confirming the negative self-evaluation. Guilt may be expressed as an excessive responsibility for some untoward or tragic event. The sense of worthlessness or guilt may be of delusional proportions.
>
> Thoughts of death or suicide are common. There may be fear of dying, the belief that the individual or others would be better off dead, wishes to die, or suicidal plans or attempts. (pp. 210–211)

The DSM–III has become an indispensable tool for insurance companies, judges and juries involved in insanity defenses, psychiatric interns and residents threading their way through chaotic emergency rooms, and anyone else who merely needs a descriptive summary of psychiatric syndromes.

While the experience of depression is *never* pleasant, depressions differ not only in their severity and degree of subjective pain, but also to the extent to which they are adaptive or maladaptive, disruptive or reparative, and in their ability to motivate the victims to change specific aspects of their lives, including their psychological defenses. How can a depression be adaptive? By that I mean that at times even a severe and long-lasting depression can be a creative, even ingenious solution to intrapsychic or interpersonal conflicts and stresses. The best example that comes to my mind of a depression being adaptive is the story of Dorothy.

DOROTHY

This cheerful, quick-witted lady was born in a small town in Arkansas at the beginning of World War I. She had grown up as a foster child who had been given to a couple of extremely stern, religious fanatics, who abused her psychologically and physically until she reached her teens. When Dorothy turned 19 she married Matt, a man who was taciturn, uncommunicative, and extremely ambitious. He, too, had been abused as a child.

Though neither of them ever spoke of their abuse to anybody—
in fact, they barely mentioned it to each other—they were determined that history should not repeat itself. They succeeded;
they never laid hands on their own three children. Matt, besides
being the town librarian, was also a dedicated historian. Whatever time was not taken up by his library duties and his various
church activities was devoted to the compilation of an enormous
treatise on the history of his county since Colonial times. He was
a loving though somewhat forbidding figure in the household
who spent very little time with the family. He was both a demanding and an absentee father. Dorothy raised her first two
children firmly and evenhandedly though not with much open
affection. Since she too spent a great deal of time in various
church activities, she expected her children to become self-
sufficient at a rather young age. They had to become earnest
little adults quite early in life. This arrangement, which in such a
religious little town was eminently socially acceptable, really
represented a working compromise formation for parents who
knew instinctively that due to the abuse they themselves had
suffered, their emotional resources were limited in the mothering department. But in this particular environment, duty to God
and the church was considered to be at least as important as the
duty to one's children. Joy in this household was defined mostly
as spiritual joy and as the pleasure one derives from a job well
done. There was next to no friction, since the entire family operated on the principle that unless you can say something good
about somebody or something, you'd better not say anything at
all. They all firmly believed in the power of positive thinking.
When Dorothy's first two children were twelve and ten respectively, Dorothy unexpectedly became pregnant again. After the
delivery of her third baby, Dorothy became sickly, morose, and
totally lacking in energy. She could not help focusing excessively
on each and every one of her physical symptoms, and she was
full of a terrible sense of dread and foreboding. Everywhere she
looked, she saw the signs of impending disaster and she was
tearful most of the time. To all intents and purposes she became

an invalid, and for the next six years she rarely left her sickbed. She taught her older children how to look after the little one and when this girl entered the first grade, Dorothy began to recover until eventually she became her old, healthy, and energetic self again. She never had another episode like this, or even one similar to it. During her "illness" she suffered from many fears, obsessional ruminations about the various aches and pains in her body, she cried when she was alone, and she felt blue most of the time. On the other hand, she was thankful for and pleased with the care she received from her family, her physician, her minister, and from her friends from church, and she was proud of the fact that her two older children so competently took care of the baby and of much of the rest of the housework. The people around her never failed to praise Dorothy for bearing her illness so stoically, her family made allowances for an occasional attack of bad temper and for her rather limited interest in her children's lives. The physician and her minister consoled her time and again when she expressed her guilt over not being able to take better care of her children and her husband. After all, they assured her, her illness was hardly her own fault. Obviously, to think of Dorothy's illness as a simple postpartum depression is far too simple, for it would not do justice to the two adaptive and reparative functions that this episode entailed. Though objectively the experience qualifies for what the DSM–III would classify as a major depression, it also served at least two vital functions in Dorothy's intrapsychic life and in her relationship with her third child: It provided her with the loving and meticulous emotional and physical care reserved for babies and invalids, thereby giving her the childhood she never had. Of equal importance was the fact that the shock she experienced when she found herself pregnant again unconsciously must have served as a signal to herself that her resources of mothering behavior had been exhausted, had been used up, by her first two babies. In its stead, a deeper layer, her capacity for child abuse threatened to emerge. Thus, a depression masked as a physical illness was economically an ingenious solution since it provided her with an opportunity for emotional refueling and at the same time it protected her from her abusive potential until that particular danger had passed. Her "illness" had not been a threat to her sense of self, to her concept of who she was as a person; those years had been very painful, but they had been God's will. Thus, the episode could easily be integrated into her ongoing biography. Given the alternative, the children fared very well, though the deficit in mothering has left its scars in varying degrees in all three of them.

For the majority of people, it seems that depression is primarily, if not exclusively, a painful event with few redeeming features. Depressions come in all different shapes and sizes, and they vary with respect to the components that caused or contributed to them:

First of all, we have to distinguish between unipolar and bipolar (manic-depressive) depression. They differ in their manifestations, including their underlying psychological and biological pathologies, and they require different therapies. Bipolar depression is a spectrum disorder. That means that people suffering from it can be in varying degrees manic or even-tempered, depressed or normal, or alternating between mania and depression. Unipolar depressives are *never* manic, though they may be what we call in common parlance a bit "hyper"; they usually are in varying degrees either even-tempered or depressed. Bipolar disorders can be mild or severe, intermittent or chronic, and they will be discussed in the second section of this chapter.

Both unipolar and bipolar depressions can be primary or secondary. A primary depression is one where the particular mood disorder *is* the dominant problem, while in a secondary depression some other factor or dysfunction, sometimes in conjunction with a number of psychological and/or social variables, produces the symptoms which we identify as depression. First of all, a depression can be secondary to some other psychiatric disorder, such as schizophrenia. Secondly, it can be "masked," which means that what we call the "presenting problem," i.e., the difficulties that the patient complains about in the first session, are symptoms such as vague somatic complaints with dysphoric, i.e., joyless mood, recurrent, destructive behavior patterns, proneness to accidents, the pursuit of polysurgery (multiple surgical procedures) in the absence of real physical complaints, certain panic states, and compulsive self-destructive habits, such as shoplifting and gambling. Thirdly, depression can be a symptom of physical illness. Mark S. Gold (1987) claims that 40% of all diagnoses of unipolar or bipolar depressions are inaccurate. Gold believes that in those instances the examining health professional or general physician failed to recognize the depressive symptoms as constituting the result of some common and some not-so-common physical ailments, and who therefore proceeded to treat the mood disorder instead of the real physical problem. While this figure strikes me as unrealistically high, it is nevertheless important to know that there are 75 distinct physical ailments that produce a clinical picture that resembles a unipolar or bipolar depression, for example: Alzheimer's disease, diabetes, AIDS, mononucleosis, heart disease, Lyme disease, thyroid disorders, viral pneumonia, lupus, multiple sclerosis, testicular and pancreatic cancer, and cancers of the spinal cord and the brain, etc. The following drugs can mimic unipolar depression: PCP (angel dust), toluene, marijuana, amphetamines, cocaine, sedative hypnotic drugs, Methadone and certain hypertensives (drugs designed to lower high blood pressure). Bipolar symptoms can be the result of the following drugs: PCP, marijuana, amphetamines, and cocaine. Extreme nutritional deficiencies can also produce depression, notably Vitamin B6, B3 (niacin, the absence of which causes pellagra) B12, folic acid, B2, B1, and vitamin C. For example, a diet without any carbohydrates would lack some specific and important amino acids, the precursors or building blocks for the chemical compound called tryptophane which, in turn, is the precursor for serotonin, an extremely important neurotransmitter chemical which is necessary for maintaining a well-functioning sleep-wake cycle. Low serotonin transmission is associated with unipolar depression and a number of other affective disorders (see the chapters on biology and psychobiology). Deficiencies in certain metals such as sodium, potassium, iron, calcium, magnesium, and zinc have also been implicated. Conversely, excess amounts of lead, mercury, arsenic, bismuth, aluminum, and bromides in the human body can result in similar symptoms. None of what has just been said should be terribly surprising, for a number of reasons: First of all, in a way, "we are what we eat," or shoot or snort or smoke or introduce into our bodies in some other fashion. The brain, like any other organ in our bodies, is dependent on specific nutrients or chemicals and it cannot function properly in the presence of some others. Secondly, a chemical imbalance in one organ system is likely to cause a chemical imbalance, even structural and functional changes, in another.

In making the distinction between primary and secondary depression, it is important to note that it is not always clear what comes first. Alcoholism in particular is a case in point and the same is probably true for other substance abuses as well. Alcoholism seems to entail several syndromes, some of which are primary, and others secondary. Alcohol can, and very often is, a form of self-medication for affective disorders. Applied over time it will produce a set of its own depressive symptoms. The example of Bernie, which will be discussed below, should illustrate that complex interrelationship.

Depressions can be latent, masked, or overt. Diagnostically, this poses a number of tricky questions, most of which will be addressed in later chapters, for example: What is the probable course of a masked or latent depression, or simply that of a depressive potential over a life-time? How universal is a depressive potential? And if it is, how useful is it then as a diagnostic entity? Put differently, is it possible—or useful—to view all psychopathology which is not depression as a defensive formation to avoid depression? For example, as I have shown elsewhere (Schad-Somers, 1982), masochism originally evolves as a defense against feeling unloved, even hated. To acknowledge the presence of parental rejection would expose the infant to the fear of abandonment, which, if it were to occur, would result in an abandonment depression. Additionally, the intrapsychic and the interpersonal dynamics operating in the masochistic individual often result in disappointment, punishment, rejection, and abandonment and, consequently, *eventually* in depression. Pathological narcissism, with all its attendant vulnerabilities in self-esteem, also always threatens the patient with the possibility of plunging into a depression. When that happens, and when the depression is severe, it becomes, for the time being, the primary problem that has to be addressed. The treatment of the character pathology then has to wait until the depression has lifted sufficiently for a further analysis of what *caused* the affective response. In order to accomplish this, a short term application of an antidepressant medication may be called for.

When I recently made a list of all my patients, past and present, who have *never* been depressed for more than a day or two, the following diagnostic categories emerged: conversion hysteria, atypical mania, a-motivational syndrome, developmental arrest, sexual perversions, and infantile and histrionic personalities. Sexual perversions are a prime example of what I would consider to be the psychological equivalent of what is known in physics as "black holes"—matter so dense that no light can penetrate. The alternative to a perversion would be a devastating depression, because so much pathology is compressed into it. For example, sexual sadomasochists, whose defensive structure is threatened before the patients are ready to give it up, will take instant flight rather than face what would amount to an incapacitating depression; or, worse yet, such an implosion of particles could easily result in psychosis. In other words, sexual sadomasochism is a disorder that can only be treated if the underlying depressive potential is avoided as much as is humanly possible.

However, while diagnostically and therapeutically it is of

vital importance to be aware of and to appreciate a patient's depressive potential, which can lie underneath many forms of character pathology, to respect it, and to time interpretations and other interventions accordingly, the distinction between overt depression and depressive potential is nevertheless a valid one. A once-in-a-lifetime major depressive episode, even untreated, can also have an important signal function in that it may alert a person to the fact that he or she has a profound vulnerability, a "depressive fault line," as it were, that makes it imperative to protect this line even at the cost of rearranging some major aspects of one's life and, at least temporarily, and/or sacrificing some precious goals or ambitions. Marianne is a perfect example of such a psychic patchwork solution.

MARIANNE

Her upbringing had been psychologically abusive, neglectful, and punctuated by several dramatic abandonments. Her parents are chronically unhappy, distrustful, and socially inept people, who had always been unable to empathize with their children's feelings. For example, when at the age of four Marianne was taken to the hospital to have her appendix removed, she was not told beforehand that anything was going to happen. Her parents simply dropped her off at the admissions office and then vanished.

Marianne, having been berated as a child, pushed away, criticized, never praised or encouraged, was therefore determined quite early in life to escape from this mean-spirited working-class environment and to make a very different life for herself. Shortly before graduating from college, she fell passionately in love with a young man who represented the very life she had envisioned for herself. It was the happiest, most glorious period in her life. However, after a year of bliss, it abruptly collapsed. Her boyfriend cheated on her, and when she confronted him, he laughed at her, giving her to believe that her claims on his love were all fantasy on her part, and treating the entire relationship as if it had been merely a casual fling. As a result, she suffered an undiagnosed and untreated major depressive episode. As she remembers it, and as her parents told her, she was almost completely incoherent, crying hysterically, and for over two weeks stayed in bed, curled up in a fetal position, not answering her phone. Eventually her parents arrived on the scene and took her to their home, where they looked after her until she recovered six months later. They did not attempt to get any professional help for her, but simply waited until the depression had run its course. For almost 20 years following this episode, Marianne had many boyfriends, but she always saw to it that she left them before she could get too involved. She finished school, obtained a graduate degree, and she built a modest, somewhat unexciting life for herself. To liven things up, she spun many dreams and fantasies, involving assorted get-rich-quick schemes, none of them really crazy, just unrealistic, given her limited funds and connections. She had many friends and several hobbies. People regarded her as shy, unassuming, somewhat lacking in ambition, mild-mannered, perhaps slightly dysphoric, and extremely sensitive to rejection and criticism. Her life seemed forever to be tinged with just a touch of quiet desperation. Marianne's favorite reading was of the escapist kind: science fiction and mysteries. She never seriously fell in love again and she also never had another depressive episode. However, to the extent that she risked exposing herself to small romantic disappointments—which was rare— she would react to them with a depression quite disproportionate to the provocation. What she experienced on those occasions were miniature versions of her original breakdown. However, unlike the first one, they only lasted anywhere from a few hours to a few days. Until she did a great deal of therapeutic work, she was a latent depressive who simply managed to avoid the *one* trauma that she knew could send her over the edge, namely abandonment and unrequited love.

What brought her to therapy was not depression at all, it

was a "romantic conflict" for which she just needed some counseling. She was seriously considering a more intense and committed relationship with her current boyfriend, who clearly wanted marriage and children. Though Marianne had some doubts about this man, he seemed decent enough, and Marianne was quite aware of the fact that her biological clock was running out. The subtext, the latent plea underneath the "counseling" request was actually: "Help me out of this mess, I have crossed the line into the danger zone." She soon did, in fact, disengage herself from this relationship and the therapeutic task, then, was to depression-proof her while avoiding a depression—essentially, to treat the mood disorder in its absence. That meant working through her mostly loveless childhood, without allowing her to plunge into total desolation; to strengthen her defenses, her coping skills, and her ability to deal with separation and abandonment. As a psychological task this can only be compared to the performance of a high-wire act without the benefit of a safety net. In this endeavor, she succeeded admirably. Given different circumstances it is quite conceivable that Marianne might have gone through adult life without ever coming face-to-face with her depressive potential, or, for that matter, into psychotherapy. There are plenty of people who structure their lives in such a way that the vulnerable core stays protected. They can lead extremely busy lives, never settle down, or, alternatively, settle down with a detached partner, devote themselves passionately to causes or hobbies, travel extensively, and eventually go to their graves vaguely contented, or discontented, as the case may be, but without the trauma of a depressive breakdown and without becoming a statistic in the incidence of depression in this country.

Before proceeding with the classification and description of the symptomatology of unipolar depression, two case histories have been chosen to illustrate concretely the history and the clinical picture of a major and primary unipolar depression: Bernie and Martha. While the designation of Bernie's depression as primary, rather than as secondary to alcohol abuse, may be arguable, for reasons that have been addressed earlier, he qualifies in my judgment for the label of primary depression.

BERNIE

Bernie was born in Austria, the only son of a wealthy merchant family who was in the process of trying to escape what his parents feared might result from a possible expansion of the Third Reich. While this foresight turned out to have been astute, it also meant that Bernie was separated from his parents on and off from a very early age. In fact, it was not until Bernie was six years old that the family reunited in New York. While the process of emigration had been a protracted nightmare, the family now settled happily into the New World. This pleasant state of affairs did not last long, however. Once the United States entered the war, Bernie's parents, who were not Jewish, felt like unwelcome, even alien, outsiders. From that time on, and to this day, they pretty much kept to themselves. Though both parents had to work to make ends meet, a great deal of time and attention on both parents' part was given to Bernie's schooling and the supervision of his homework.

Bernie, in looking back, remembered feeling that he was being groomed for the position of family ambassador to the outside world, one that his parents dared not enter. Whether or not Bernie's parents had always been as withdrawn and reclusive as Bernie remembers them is hard to tell. All we know is that in America they never became acculturated, they merely transported the Vienna of the 1920s to New York of the 1940s and 50s, though without the trimmings of wealth that they had enjoyed in Europe. Bernie grew up, living a bilingual and bicultural life, plotting his escape from this dreary, monotonous home where nobody ever really had fun. He did so by getting excellent grades and by applying for scholarships to Ivy League schools. He won a scholarship to Yale and eventually earned a

Ph.D. in English literature. He began to teach at a college, and to write fiction, and those were probably the happiest years of his life.

However, when an expected promotion did not materialize, due to a lack of scholarly publications on Bernie's part, he decided to "think things over" for a while. In order to pay his rent, Bernie got a hack license, drove a cab just often enough to get by, and began to write his first major novel. This temporary arrangement gradually became a permanent one, not through any conscious decision on Bernie's part, but simply because he had managed somehow to suspend the dimension of time in his life. His wants were few: a simple apartment in Greenwich Village, ample time to write, a beat-up Smith-Corona and a circle of like-minded literary friends. The neighborhood bar became a regular meeting place for his group—though Bernie could be just as happy as a solitary patron, drinking quietly, thinking, observing, and taking mental notes of things around him. During those years there was also a series of girlfriends, all of whom, judging from his descriptions, seemed interchangeable in their personalities. They were earnest young women, seeking careers in the world of literature, and they were all well-spoken, ambitious, and attractive. As Bernie grew older, his girlfriends became younger. He kept regular, though superficial contact with his parents, who grew increasingly more reclusive. He joined them once every couple of weeks for that Central European institution known as "coffee and cake" which can occupy an entire afternoon, but must definitely end before dinner. He kept these time-limited engagements with his parents until they retired to Florida.

On the whole, his had been a fairly contented existence. His friends never failed to praise his short stories and book-length manuscripts, his involvements with women had never been intense enough to make the breakup a dramatic event—these women seemed to have just faded away—every couple of years he submitted a manuscript or two to a publisher, and they were usually returned with the standard rejection slip, "interesting, but not appropriate for us at this time," and he placed a few short stories in some of the more obscure literary quarterlies. He bore the rejection slips with equanimity; but then, very little upset this mild-mannered, roly-poly man who, with his bulky sweaters and his mop of grey hair, resembled a teddy bear. When he was 47 years old, a woman he had been living with for five years abruptly left him. Only, instead of fading away, she vented her full fury over his passivity, lack of ambition, and his unwillingness to commit himself to a more serious and ongoing relationship. This tirade shook him up much more than he admitted to himself at that time.

During that same year Bernie had sent his very first novel, his youthful masterpiece, to the editor for whom he had had the most respect. After six months, the editor returned it with a rejection letter so full of contempt, so scathing, its bile content would have seemed potent enough to shred 20 manuscripts. From that point on Bernie, who had always been a regular and serious drinker, began to drink in earnest, consuming at least half a quart of vodka per day. Although previously he had been a quiet drinker, he now became increasingly boisterous, even belligerent, not infrequently provoking fights in the seedy bars he now visited. While his autonomic nervous system seems to have somehow remembered how to drive a cab well enough not to get into an accident, the sight of a blank page in his typewriter now produced total paralysis in his brain. His self-esteem was split into two opposing parts: a self-proclaimed genius at night, and a useless, despicable old drunk in the morning. After several years of this, the cab-driving began to take its toll—his back protested. The family physician prescribed Valium to ease what he presumed to be muscle spasms. Bernie liked this prescription a lot since it helped not only his back, but his growing insomnia as well. On the day Bernie turned 50, he engaged one of his passengers, an attractive English major attending Barnard College, in a conversation about literary careers. When he looked into the rearview mirror for her facial response to the tale of his life, he expected, if not admiration, at least interest. Instead, what he saw was pity and even contempt. After having dropped off his passenger, Bernie hit the bar nearest Columbia University and proceeded to alternate shots of vodka with 5 mgs of Valium until the bartender there, "who has seen it all," anticipated the impending disaster and called an ambulance. The hospital pumped Bernie's stomach, stabilized his respiration, kept him for observation overnight, and sent him home the next morning with a prescription for a tricyclic antidepressant medication and the advice that he should join AA.

MARTHA

Martha, who was born a year before Dorothy—that is, a year before World War I—grew up in a world that was very different from Dorothy's small-town Arkansas. Martha's father was a well-known physicist, and Martha grew up in a world of scholarship for which the University of Chicago was renowned. While her father was the scholarly paterfamilias, her mother had established for herself a small reputation as a semiprofessional musician. It seems that as a family unit they all functioned as extensions of the famous father. Much of the child care, therefore, was given over to servants. In addition, Martha's father employed his wife as an honorary teaching assistant who had to attend all his lectures and seminars, leaving her even less time for the children. Martha's parents expected that their three children would follow in their footsteps, and they barely managed to hide their profound disappointment when the two younger ones showed no inclination in that direction. Worse, shortly before the oldest child completed his Ph.D. dissertation in philosophy, he was killed in a car crash.

The mother mourned the death of her oldest child and only son profoundly. In fact, it seems, in retrospect, that she suffered a fairly intense depressive episode, coupled with melancholia, that lasted for several years. When she emerged from it, she had rejoined the Catholic church, an affiliation she had dropped when she married her husband, who was a devout agnostic. During that time, Martha, who had dropped out of college in her second year, became a very junior staff member at an avant garde literary magazine. Shortly thereafter, and to everybody's surprise, she met and married Robert, a businessman 12 years her senior. They moved to New York and, within four years, Martha gave birth to a son and two daughters, becoming a suburban full-time housewife and mother. After five years of happiness the marriage began to turn rocky. Though the couple never formally separated, husband and wife nevertheless had prolonged separations due first to Robert's wartime service and, later, because he started a business in Florida which he sold after three years. Even though he returned to New York, he continued to travel extensively, leaving for weeks at a time. In that fashion, Robert could play out his ambivalence towards his wife without having to state it openly; he could simply point to external circumstances. In a similar vain, Martha, who was an unusually reserved and proud woman, could save face, overlook the mistresses, maintain a facade of a happy marriage and attribute her periods of listlessness and irritability towards her children to the fact that she spent so much time with her husband away on business.

Martha never really gave up the pursuit of her intellectual ambitions; rather, she put them on the back burner. Not knowing whether or not the marriage would endure, and sensing that autonomous pursuits on her part could constitute the straw that would break this marital camel's back, she let things ride. Also, Robert, not unlike Martha's father, had become the family icon who encouraged autonomy among the members of his family *as long as* it did not impinge on his pampered status as paterfamilias. Furthermore, when her older children were already in their teens, Martha became pregnant again. After the youngest daughter was born, the marriage became much more stable, though not less volatile. Robert travelled less and less and, after the first signs of cardiac trouble, pretty much gave it up altogether. Besides, Martha, too, became increasingly concerned with her physical health. She suffered from a variety of ailments, none of them really incapacitating, but serious enough to require major surgery and some resulting in major and permanent dietary restrictions.

When Martha was in her early 50s the following events took place in the span of only six months. One of her children got married and moved away; another left for Europe; and the third went off to study in Japan. Last, but by no means least, Robert died unexpectedly. This came as a complete shock; Martha felt totally unprepared for widowhood. It had been Robert who had been the extrovert in this marriage. It was he who brought people into the house, while it was Martha who often functioned as the inhibitor of his at times too-expansive hospitality. Also, as long as the older children still lived at home, they filled the house with their own friends. Predictably, then, after Robert's funeral, Martha and her youngest child found themselves in a house that was far too empty and far too quiet. Three years after Robert's death, both of Martha's parents, with whom she had remained extremely close, died within six months of each other. Besides the losses due to death, and her children leaving home, and the loss of a social network that had been maintained by her family, without her having to take any initiative, Martha now also had to come to terms with losses of a more personal kind: menopause, and the experience of increasing immobility due to bouts with arthritis. Furthermore, some of her chronic physical conditions having onset prior to Robert's death became more serious, with more frequent episodes. In the course of three years she turned from a lively matron into an elderly, ailing, lonely widow, a woman who felt she had nothing to look forward to.

Shortly after Robert's death she had announced that she was planning to commit suicide on the precise day she reached the age that Robert had been when he died, i.e., 12 years later. Her family, concerned both with her declining physical health and her deepening depression, expressed worry but did not take any decisive action. Twelve years later, when the appointed time arrived, Martha planned a trip to Europe to visit one of her children. She made these plans in spite of the fact that she was suffering from a bout of phlebitis. When her children pointed out to her that such a trip presented an excellent opportunity to "accidentally" die en route, she brushed this off as absurd and confirmed her travel plans.

As it turned out, she had a good trip. However, as her physical ailments, particularly her arthritis, worsened, threatening her with the prospect of total immobility, her internist recommended replacement surgery for two of her joints. When she arrived at the hospital for special surgery, however, she was too ill to be admitted and was transferred to a general hospital nearby. She was clearly very ill and profoundly depressed. However, months and months of testing and observation did not disclose an organic cause for this "failure to thrive" syndrome. Finally she got well enough to be discharged, and the physician in charge recommended psychotherapy, a course of action she would not even consider.

Upon her return home, Martha felt worse again, lost interest in food, in people, in books—even in her cats. She thought and talked about suicide and death constantly, and eventually she succeeded in convincing one of her children that since she was suffering from terminal cancer it would be an act of filial love and mercy to provide her with the drugs necessary to end her life. During those months she spent most of her time in bed, her demeanor was either stony or frantic; she stopped being weepy, but became incoherent at times, slipping occasionally into psychosis. By the same token, if it became necessary, she could become her old rational self again.

The child who had arranged for the drugs informed the others of their mother's impending death from cancer and arranged good-bye visits. As it turned out, none of the plans came off. The drugs ended up at the bottom of Lake Michigan. From that point on, Martha began to recover. She slowly but steadily regained her mental and physical health, and underwent replacement surgery as well as physical therapy and rehabilitation. She found freelance editorial work, which she enjoyed immensely and for which she was uniquely talented, and her depression has vanished completely. The subject was never discussed. It became a non-event. Nothing happened.

Unipolar, primary depression (single-episode, intermittent, or chronic) is probably several disorders, but at the very least we must distinguish between two different types of it. The literature on the subject, the different schools of thought, have used different terms and different criteria to distinguish between them: autonomous (melancholia) vs. reactive depression; endogenous vs. psychogenic; psychotic vs. neurotic, and vital vs. neurotic. To complicate matters even further, use of these terms has changed over the years. However, despite these somewhat confusing designations, these distinctions refer to some very real and very important dimensions of depressions and/or patient populations: namely (1) ability to experience pleasure when a pleasurable event occurs; (2) response to psychosocial interventions; (3) whether or not precipitating psychological events were present or absent; and (4) whether or not there is delusional thinking or psychosis. What these dichotomies intuitively and accurately try to capture is *the extent to which more or less autonomous biological processes* predominate in the picture. As will be shown in the subsequent chapters on biology and psychobiology, we now have solid empirical biological evidence that such factors do indeed exist. In terms of genetic biology, we even know what biological marker they are near, namely dysfunctions in the hypothalamic-pituitary-adrenal system (HPA), as well as that of sleep patterns (REM latencies) (for details, see Chapter 5).

However, the relative weight or importance of these biological-genetic factors does not necessarily determine the severity of a depression. Both endogenomorphic depressions and neurotic ones represent a spectrum of diversity as well as severity, with the neurotic group being the more heterogeneous. In 1974 Donald Klein proposed the following distinction between vital (endogenomorphic) and neurotic (nonendogenomorphic) depression, arguing that vital depressions result from an inhibited or unresponsive pleasure center, while neurotic depressions arise from the inability to tolerate frustration. Klein's schema has had two advantages over all the previous models or dichotomies: It recognizes two types of the disorder, and it proposes a psychological theory for each, because, additionally, Klein suggests a number of attitudinal variables to connect the presumed cause, namely inhibited pleasure centers, or the inability to tolerate frustration, with the manifest symptoms, such as hopelessness, lack of interest, guilt, agitation, etc. Klein argues that an impaired pleasure center means an impairment of a person's reward system, while the inability to tolerate frustration interferes with the ability to deal with stress. Examples for intervening variables in the case of neurotic depression are: anticipation of pleasure and pain and their relative distribution, demoralization, and low self-esteem. For vital depressions he lists the following: cognitive impairments pertaining to cognition and information processing, difficulties with learning, concentration and memory, and varying degrees of psychomotor retardation or agitation.

Whether one accepts Klein's model or not, subsequent research has upheld the validity of a distinction between depressions that are predominantly endogenomorphic and those that are primarily nonendogenomorphic depressions. (Willner 1985). The endogenomorphic group is characterized by the following characteristics, which consist of clusters of variables: (1) *pleasure:* these people are less talented for and less inclined towards the pursuit of pleasurable experiences, they perceive themselves as being deficient in that department, they are not good at finding alternatives if one source of pleasure is cut off, they typically have poor social skills, and, to make matters worse, nondepressed people tend to avoid them, for they make poor company; (2) *pain:* depressed patients rate unpleasant or stressful events as more painful than normal controls, they get more upset by them, and they are more vulnerable to negative social reactions, such as disagreements, criticism, or to being ignored. Information processing and memory are biased in the direction of the frequency and the severity of negative events and their meaning; (3) *attitudes:* self-esteem is generally low, they perceive themselves as helpless, not in control of their environment and, at the same time, they feel inordinately responsible for it. They tend to be introverts, rather than extroverts, a trait that seems to be related, biologically, to the impairment in the HPA system.

Paul Willner, who uses the terms endogenomorphic versus nonendogenomorphic, has pointed out that there two principal sources of well-being for humans: (1) Anticipation of future rewards; and (2) actual satisfaction and fulfillment of wished-for pleasures which then result in behavioral quiescence. Klein refers to these two entities as the "hunt," or the "chase," and the "feast." Consequently, it would make sense that the impairment of either would have a corresponding form of depression. Endogenomorphic depression is characterized by an insensitivity to rewards and, consequently, lack of incentive or motivation. It has an autonomous course. Melancholics, as endogenomorphic depressives are also called, are typically unresponsive to attempts at consolation and comfort. Because of this dysfunction in the reward system in the brain, alleviating the conditions that precipitated the depression does not spell relief, or even improvement. The nonendogenomorphic depressive finds no rewards, has no skills to get them, is anxious and hostile, but responds well to attention and reassurance. These individuals form a part of a spectrum of pathological conditions which, among others, include alcoholism, drug dependence, and personality disorders. The latter, in turn, probably represent alternate outcomes of a common underlying pathology. Nonendogenomorphic depression can range in its severity and manifestations from neurotic to psychotic.

While this distinction between two types of unipolar depression represents an important *theoretical* differentiation, it does not, in reality, occur very often in a pure form. There are several reasons. First of all, the two syndromes are not mutually exclusive; on the contrary, they tend to reinforce each other. The patient suffering from endogenomorphic depression tends to act in ways which induce the people in his or her environment to withdraw support. Conversely, the nonendogenomorphic's failure to find love and affection acts as a chronic uncontrollable stress, an important causative factor in endogenomorphic depression. In other words, what we encounter in reality are always mixed types, which only differ with respect to the relative distribution of autonomous and reactive variables.

What the concept of mutual reinforcement of these two types of depression hints at, but does not yet spell out, is the element of time, i.e., the notion that personality and psychopathology are continuous processes, structures that can and do change over time, sometimes for the better, sometimes for the worse. In other words, the time element alone suggests that, diagnostically, we have to distinguish between specific depressions and the depression-prone person. Martha's depressions started in her early 30s. Back then they were mild and intermittent. In her 50s the picture changed dramatically to severe and chronic, culminating in a major depression in her 60s and then, seemingly inexplicably, it went into a complete remission which lasted through her 70s.

Marianne, in contrast, had one major depressive episode in her 20s, leaving a remnant of mild, intermittent dysphoria; while Bernie showed signs of a mild but chronic masked depression, with moderate-to-heavy drinking patterns through his 40s, and finally evolved into a case of full-fledged secondary alcoholism. In combination they resulted in a major depression.

These three very different lines of development are reflections of the variants of human demoralization or encouragement. What saved Dorothy from succumbing to her abusive childhood we will never know. Her first major crisis in adult life, her postpartum "illness," turned out to be a creative and successful solution, one which helped strengthen her self-confidence rather than diminishing it. Since the major source of interpersonal satisfaction had been her fellow church members, the growing up and the marriages of her children spelled relief rather than loss. In fact, when Matt died, two years after their retirement in Florida, Dorothy came truly into her own. Due to Matt's extreme miserliness, she found herself a well-to-do widow who happily joined what Znaiecky-Lopata (1973) has called the "community of widows." She enjoys spending money, visiting her children, traveling abroad, and being the sole mistress of her own life. Having gotten a more than passing grade for each successive phase of development in her adult life has had a positive cumulative effect, thereby giving her an additional boost to her pride and self-esteem.

Martha, in contrast, received very few of these encouragements along the way. Instead, she experienced more and more uncontrollable stresses. To even imagine that she had any control over Robert's marital ambivalence would have bordered on delusional thinking. What is more, it left no room for negotiating a more equitable relationship. Though Robert was mostly a benign tyrant, he was a tyrant nevertheless. Martha not only tolerated the infidelities, she concluded that voluntary submission to the will of another person was, by definition, not really submission. While she accomplished her major goal—the marriage lasted—the process itself had many demoralizing features, all her rationalizations notwithstanding. After Robert's death the succession of losses proved overwhelming. Life had become very lonely and empty. She had no faith or religion to comfort her. Only half in jest did she once remark wistfully: "Too bad, I have talent for religion," a stance which is entirely in keeping with her critical mind. Furthermore, Martha had little experience with initiating friendships and, given her lack of formal education and training, she could not imagine any kind of employment that could possibly have been congruent with her intelligence and knowledge. Her physical ailments, particularly her arthritis, meant becoming an invalid, a helpless cripple.

With each loss and each year, she lost more of what little self-esteem she had had to begin with, until eventually she could think of absolutely nothing that would appreciably improve her life. All she could see was a progressive deterioration, with no relief. Suicide, indeed, seemed to be the only affirmative action left to her. Besides, it was a major challenge to her manipulative skills to have it done for her and to make it look like a natural death.

For Marianne, one major demoralizing experience in her 20s all but overwhelmed her. In the course of it she lost all power over all the different dimensions of her life, an experience that proved to have been sufficiently traumatic for her to lower all her ambitions, romantically and professionally. Life was safe, though not terribly exciting for almost the next two decades, at the end of which she was ready to fall in love again. Once she started expanding her life, branching out and trying new options, encouragement fed on encouragement, and she is now full of hope and confidence.

Bernie evolved in the opposite direction: After his first disappointment, a faculty position which, quite predictably, was not forthcoming, he settled into a fairly comfortable state of chronic low-level depression cushioned by a daily dose of vodka. It was only in the three years preceding his suicide attempt that the succession of failures resulted in alcoholism and, correspondingly, a major depression. His self-esteem progressively eroded. Each bar-room brawl, each hangover, the continuation of his writer's block—all contributed to further intensify his self-loathing. Being treated like an abysmal failure by his last girlfriend made matters worse; the contempt on the part of the one editor he valued above all others; and, finally, the horror on the part of a young undergraduate student turned out to be the straw that finally broke the camel's back. On his birthday binge, Bernie experienced himself essentially as helpless, but *not* as hopeless, since a public suicide attempt is hardly a sign of giving up. It merely indicated that Bernie thought that help could be found somewhere, other than in his own self or in his immediate circumstances and resources. Unfortunately, his vision of psychiatric care was derived from literature, or rather from the wrong novels, which clearly bore no resemblance to the reality of Bellevue Hospital. Still, he was far from giving up.

Mania is not simply the other side of the depressive coin, though, subjectively, the initial experience of the switch into mania may well feel that way: the mood is expansive, euphoric, elated or, alternatively, irritated, enraged, even homicidal. The patient is flying high, moves, thinks, and speaks rapidly; the need for sleep diminishes, and possibilities for thought or deed seem unlimited. Normal self-esteem slips into grandiosity and the vulnerability to criticism and frustration can be so extreme that reactions to the frustrating object may easily turn violent. Concentration and memory are impaired, but the manic feels compelled to pursue his or her unrealistic, even dangerous goals without interference from anybody. Manics often appear flamboyant or bizarre, overdressed or disheveled, but whatever their appearance, they are dramatic and they are on stage. In a full-blown attack of mania the victim may buy anything, be it the entire line of Perry Ellis fashion at Bloomingdale's or the Empire State Building. The manic may engage in compulsive sexual activity, shoplifting, go on binges of any kind, end up in jail, or attempt suicide. If the manic episode progresses, if it becomes more intense or pronounced, the patient may lose contact with reality, hallucinate, and become openly psychotic. The worst possible clinical picture is that of mania coupled with paranoia. For example, Dr. I. Aiken, father of the poet Conrad Aiken, was a manic-depressive who became consumed by suspicions regarding his wife's fidelity. After years of heaping accusations on her, he finally kept her up an entire night, questioning her, at the end of which, just when the sun came up, he shot and killed her, and then killed himself.

While the patient experiences the onset of mania as distinctly pleasurable, the intermediary stage is characterized by intense excitement which is thrilling and frightening at the same time. If the mania is not alleviated pharmacologically at that point, the patient will spin out of control. Though this third phase can be intensely painful, the patient can no longer bring himself to care what happens. By that time the mania has become a psychic avalanche, unstoppable and highly destructive. While patients in stage two still have a choice, either to try to control the episode by themselves, to increase the medication, or to hospitalize themselves, they are typically disinclined to exercise that option because the thrill of acute mania is too tempting. Additionally, in the course of their lives, bipolar patients experience a great deal of discouragement and demoralization due to the fact that commonly the disorder is recurrent. Seeming victories can crumple in matter of hours, with little warning, and a life that has been carefully rebuilt over the course of several years can fall apart in the course of a week. Thus, in the grip of a manic attack, a patient may easily reason, "My life's gone to hell in a basket, there's nothing left that's worth protecting anyway, but at least *this experience* feels alive and real." Furthermore, when patients return to a more normal state, they then have to face all the social, economic, and interpersonal consequences of their mania, which can be extremely shameful; so shameful, in fact, that hospitalization and suicide appear attractive by comparison.

While, on the whole, bipolar patients are a much more homogeneous group than unipolar ones, there are nevertheless major differences between them. The majority of people suffering from bipolar disorders experience in varying degrees both mania and depression. They alternate, or "cycle," as it is called, either rapidly—moment-to-moment, or frequently, as a matter of weeks or months, or only a few times over the course of their lives. Some experience long stretches of tranquillity between episodes, others are tossed back and forth continuously between these two feeling states. While an intense, acute attack of mania is almost impossible to misdiagnose—it raises gooseflesh on those who are its target—a mild case of mania can be stimulating for its recipients and pleasurable for the patient. In fact, whether mild mania is considered a problem, in need of treatment, may well depend on who looks at it.

William, for example, who at least until now, only experienced the mildly manic end of the spectrum, is a man of the most extraordinary appetites. Everything is consumed or done to excess: food, work, drink, sex, betting, gambling, bookmaking, drugs, and making money. Since, so far, his physiology matches his appetites, he seems to have the constitution of an elephant, together with a work ethic worthy of a Calvinist—an all-night orgy, with multiple partners and multiple substances has yet to keep him from getting up at six in the morning and from putting in a full day of work. He has not only gotten away with it, but he also raised several families and he has prospered. However, when one of his grown children attempted to imitate his life-style, she quickly came to grief; her drug habits were about to ruin her life. Now, with respect to the diagnosis: The therapist who is treating the *daughter*, sees an addicted family evenly divided between addicts and enablers; the psychopharmacologist who treats her also sees several generations of bipolar disorder; and this therapist, who is treating the *father*, sees a man in need of protection from his thrill-seeking behavior, as well as from his depressive potential, and to guide him safely through a midlife crisis. As will be shown in Chapter nine, the treatment plan for the family as a whole was primarily determined by what types of insights they could accept at any given point in treatment, and therefore, what types of interventions they were amenable to, rather than by what, diagnostically, the DSM–III might have suggested.

The converse, a patient who only experiences the depressive end of the spectrum, can appear equally innocuous and seemingly indistinguishable from the norm. Karl, who after many years of therapeutic work and simply astounding amounts of progress, finally put his life in order: graduate degree, job, friends, and hobbies. He nevertheless settled into a permanent state of vague discontent and anhedonia, with a teutonic appreciation for and revelry in the tragic side of life. Though he joked about it, "his dedication to being miserable," as he called it, the people around him, who have known him for years, saw Karl essentially as a "sad sack," a perpetual loser by choice and inclination. For many years he adjudicated further therapeutic work as useless. Given the fact that he would not even *consider* the possibility of trying medication, this therapist had to agree with him. Once he changed his mind, however, a minimal amount of Lithium and six more months of therapy produced what looks like a veritable miracle: a cheerful, glowing Karl, ready to live his life joyfully and energetically. Needless to say, the fact that so little medication accomplished so much was only possible because, psychodynamically, all the important pieces, necessary to really live life, were already firmly in place; they just needed a jump-start, and some fuel. The Lithium simply removed the depressive millstone that had hung around his neck for so long.

Most bipolar patients, unfortunately, are not that lucky, in that the bipolar involvement is so small. Severe manic-depressives are much more troubled by the biological component. The stories of Mary and Liz illustrate this.

MARY

When Mary, a nurse-receptionist, first presented herself, she told a very strange tale indeed. This endearing picture of the proverbial Irish charm looked like the president of a Midwestern church bazaar, or rather, as I imagine, what Dorothy must have looked like when she was her age. She had been in therapy for several years with a man who, according to her, was "a wonderful therapist," who had helped her "a great, great deal," and he had effected "a thousand percent improvement." Unfortunately, she told me, two weeks previously she had become unreasonably angry with this man, and some of his office furniture went flying. After some probing on my part, she also conceded that his glasses had been broken in the scuffle. He terminated her therapy immediately, and her therapy group had then given her a delightful farewell party, champagne and all, congratulated her on all the progress she had made, and sent her on her way. So, here she was, ready and eager to resume psychotherapy. From the way she described her previous treatment it became clear that this therapist had been determined to cure her, to get to the psychodynamic roots of her problems by aggressively pursuing her memories of family violence, a possibly incestuous relationship with a brother, by insisting on fatherly physical contact with this frightened virgin, such as hugging and holding hands, and finally by asking Mary's mother to join them in some of Mary's sessions, in order to "prove" to her that she, Mary's mother, did in fact love her.

Before agreeing to see Mary as a patient, I wanted to call her former therapist in order to get a better idea of what actually took place. Her story simply sounded too bizarre to be true. However, her former therapist not only confirmed everything that Mary had reported, he also reiterated over and over again what "a lovely, lovely girl" she had been, and what a treat it would be to get her as a patient. Furthermore, he also volunteered the information that about six months prior to her outburst of rage Mary had been given a complete psychiatric workup that showed no biological involvement, except for some depression. The element of depression had then been treated with tricyclic antidepressant medication. Since in the course of several months the tricyclic had accomplished absolutely nothing, he had suggested she discontinue it.

Clearly this man had rushed in where angels fear to tread. Furthermore, the fact that he, the therapist himself, saw no contradiction between his characterization of "such a lovely girl" and the fact that she had been so violent towards him that he had to discontinue seeing her; the fact that she had been dismissed, but that the dismissal called for a champagne send-off, suggested that the interaction itself had probably done a good job of driving Mary mad. Though Mary was clearly disturbed in a very profound way, there was nothing immediately alarming about her current symptomatology. In addition, looking at her history, she revealed signs of genius in the art of survival: (1) She had found a boss who was singularly supportive and protective of her, who always patiently counseled her, who, when she was too unhappy or distraught, personally drove her to her therapist, who tailored her work hours around her college schedule, in short, a man who effectively functioned as a cross between a parent, a nursemaid, and an adjunct therapist. Not only had Mary managed to find such an unusual man in the first place, she also continued to work for him for what by then amounted to 10 years. (2) Though while she had had a rather rough time in her mid-20s, following her father's death, when Mary became extremely overweight, and did not work but lived by her wits, she also never had a real breakdown. (3) Instead of being devastated by the experience of being thrown out of psychotherapy, she managed to resume treatment in less than two weeks. As a matter of fact, several months prior to that violent episode, when she probably sensed that something indeed was about to go very wrong in her current treatment, she decided to go window-shopping for a possible replacement. She attended a workshop offered by a feminist psychotherapy group given by a local university. She had a wonderful time and she walked away with a set of names and phone numbers, "just in case."

A precise diagnosis of the exact nature of Mary's problems seemed not possible at that time. She was, after all, at that point, a well-functioning individual, exhibiting very little *overt* psychopathology. In terms of observable behavior, including her account of her violent episode, it was far from clear what was symptomatic for the underlying disorder and what had been induced by the therapeutic interaction. What this means is the following: with a mixed picture such as this, only time can tell whether one is dealing with a latent "schizoaffective disorder" (APA, 1987) or a latent manic-depressive. As far as Mary's background was concerned, she told very little. Mary was the youngest of four children of what had once been a well-to-do family, but had become increasingly impoverished as time went on. Mary's account of her childhood years were very sketchy. She described her family as "crazy," her mother as confusing and as "crazy-making," and her father as a loving man, an alcoholic given to violent rages and physical violence. She herself was never the target of that violence—her brother was—but the task of calling the police to intervene typically fell to Mary. These incidents were never discussed, they were papered over with upper-middle-class Catholic righteousness—massive denial. Mary hinted at a sexual involvement with her brother during her teens but she refused to talk about that. (This experience turned out to be a hallucination, a not uncommon occurrence among bipolar youngsters.)

Mary began with a twice-weekly therapy schedule, all bright and new and shiny, with a great deal of enthusiasm, and she made it clear from the beginning that she could hardly wait for the time when she would be ready to also begin group therapy. She told me time and again how much she had loved her group. This made a great deal of sense. Except for her mother and a somewhat senile aunt, Mary had broken off all contact with her family, she seemed to have very few friends or acquaintances, and she was simply lonely. At the end of her first year with me, she became a member of one of my groups, where she very quickly endeared herself to all of the other members because of her charm, seeming innocence, extraordinary insights into the unconscious of others, and a complete absence of guile on her part. For the next four years therapeutic work progressed very well by focusing almost exclusively on Mary's day-to-day problems, her career aspirations, social life, school work, etc. Attending college was crucial to her happiness. The fantasy of at some point actually becoming a child therapist seemed so wonderful a future to her, that in exchange she was quite willing to forget the traumas of her childhood, to make peace with it all. The prospect of working with disturbed children seemed to be more than sufficient compensation.

At the end of her fourth year of work with me she finally lost the one relative she had been genuinely close to, her aunt, who died after a prolonged illness. Following that loss, Mary's mother was diagnosed as having breast cancer. She was treated with surgery and radiation. It became clear to Mary that soon she would be all alone in the world. Up until that point Mary's focus had been on *keeping out* an intrusive and crazy-making family. Now she felt that they, the family, were abandoning *her*. From that point on, Mary became an increasingly difficult patient, less focused, needier, more demanding, stubborn, abrasive, and like a terrier with a bone, she worried some group incident that had happened during the previous summer.

That incident eventually revealed itself as having been Mary's first psychotic episode; no wonder she could not let go of the notion that it could be somehow righted, if only she could get an acknowledgment that it had happened, and if she also could get at least *some* revenge. Then it would all be undone, as if it had never happened. Alternatively, she thought, if she could figure out what that incident had evoked in *her*, in terms of unconscious memories and connections, the experience of a transient psychosis would then also dissolve. In her individual sessions, this became a persistent theme from September until the following May, when she began to slip into a full-fledged manic-depressive psychosis. Though she was given optimal doses of the drugs most appropriate for treating this set of symptoms, namely Lithium, Tegretol, and Navane, as much as she could be given without inducing toxicity, Mary still barely managed to stay out of a hospital for the next 18 months. Those were terrible months; she turned into a holy terror, capable of exquisite forms of sadism, malevolence, gutter language, tyrannizing her therapist with up to 25 phone calls per day, writing obscene letters, sending alarming and usually untruthful telegrams, showing up unannounced, banging on the office door, letting out bloodcurdling screams in the office as well as out in the street right under my office windows, and threatening suicide in just about every communication. She showed no mercy.

Given these problems, she left the group for two years, though she kept in close contact with all group members individually. Her individual sessions were increased from two per week to three. When this therapist ran out of steam, the psychopharmacologist took over as her psychotherapist until she was able to exercise better control over her acting-out behavior. In spite of it all, Mary managed to stay in school, continued to earn A's in her courses, and did an adequate job at work. Though she was psychotic much of the time, and in spite of the fact that she heard voices, she nevertheless succeeded in concealing that fact from everybody except her two therapists. Unfortunately, during that time she also had the opportunity to pursue an entirely unrealistic real-estate deal. In spite of the fact that she was told by everybody that she would lose her shirt, she proceeded. This cost her her entire inheritance from her beloved aunt, it cost her her apartment and, if her boss had not volunteered to bring in his own lawyer to bail her out, things would have been worse yet. As it was, she had now lost her financial security, the money that she had counted on to see her through college, working only 20–30 hours per week instead of the usual 40.

Mary seemed to be in control of her actions—for example, she never phoned when she knew that one of her fellow group members had an individual therapy session. That meant that she had to keep track of the therapy schedules of eight other people in order to conceal her "craziness." When some of them changed appointment times and thus had their sessions interrupted, she was furious with me. She simply could not comprehend the fact that the real point was not phoning at all. In that sense she was not in control. The psychotic steam had to blow off somewhere, and she chose what seemed to her to be the safest place: the therapy situation. Her rage at her therapist was also based on the at-times powerful delusion that the therapist *was* the illness and had to be fought at all costs. This presented a difficult dilemma, wanting to kill what she knew to be her lifeline, to rid herself of her madness without losing the important other: a delicate balance indeed.

LIZ

Liz's first contact with me was also rather unusual. She phoned to introduce herself and she announced that she had just been thrown out by her latest therapist—her tenth as it turned out—and that this therapist had tossed my book on sadomasochism in her direction with the remark, "You are so sick, people even write books about the likes of you." Liz had read the book from cover to cover and she was in full agreement with her former therapist's appraisal: She felt that she was indeed the quintessential sadomasochist, mostly at the sadistic end of the spectrum, and she was quite proud of that fact. Consequently, she argued, I would be the ideal therapist for her. The 44-year-old woman who appeared the following day was overweight, unkempt, dressed in a style best described as "construction worker special" and, most disturbingly, she was for the most part toothless. She was also extremely articulate, intelligent, and psychologically astute. She indicated that she was a successful psychotherapist in private practice.

Liz managed to cram more information into this first 45-minute session than most patients accomplish in six months. Her family life had been extremely chaotic, her father had been explosive and often violent, while she described her mother as provocative. Though the family was rather poor, they felt that it was their Christian duty to adopt two children—orphans—in addition to their own two. Liz had had one breakdown at age 19. No specific diagnosis was given, as far as Liz could remember, except that the attending psychiatrist informed her parents upon admission that Mary probably would have to be hospitalized for the rest of her life. As it turned out, her hospital stay was extremely short; within less than a couple of weeks she resumed her life as secretarial student. Soon thereafter, she got married. After the birth of her second child, Mary had another breakdown, requiring another brief stay in a mental hospital.

Following discharge, she discovered her lesbianism and she became politically active. Consequently, she left her family and entered various consciousness-raising groups. She became involved in a radical lesbian therapy group, first as a patient and, eventually, without the benefit of any higher education, as a practicing therapist herself. She entered college, but dropped out after a few years because her last therapist had interpreted her desire to pursue a B.A. degree as a hostile and competitive act, aimed at her therapist, who already had a B.A. With that particular therapist she became embroiled in a transference/countertransference psychosis of such intensity that Liz became acutely suicidal. In order to keep her hospitalization a secret, she committed herself under an assumed name. Within three days' time she felt well enough to leave, call for an appointment, resume her life, and enter psychotherapy again. As far as Liz was concerned, her principal problem was not ordinary psychopathology but her vulnerability towards *being driven crazy*. In fact, during her last therapeutic encounter her therapist's competitiveness, and the mystification of those feelings by calling them something other than what they really were, had "driven" her into the habit of wrist-slashing to the point where she felt it was necessary always to wear long-sleeved shirts or sweaters to hide her scars. In reality they were almost invisible, but to her they were the living proof of her vulnerability and, consequently, her victimization.

Given that estimation of her problems, she began therapy with the following prescription for her treatment: She was to be allowed to regress in order to relive her childhood traumas in a benign, all-loving environment. Empathy should replace criticism. Empathy, in her definition or interpretation of the concept, meant unconditional love and acceptance of all her utterances and actions. What she thought she needed was an "expressive psychotherapy" within the theoretical framework of what is called "Self Psychology" (Kohut, 1971, 1977). Any suggestion of behavioral controls belonged to that category of forces that had driven her crazy in the first place. Moreover, since her exhibitionistic needs had not been met during the appropriate time in childhood, the therapist now had to provide what was missing—"to admire her toes," as Liz put it. The idea was that instead of focusing on her having bounced yet another check, she should be praised for having maintained a checkbook in the first place, and had done so in spite of the fact that her family had never taught her anything having to do with money. Admonishing her for her fiscal mess was an attempt to deliberately humiliate her.

Diagnostically, what stood out, besides her mood swings and her tumultuous relationships with people, were her extreme vulnerability to criticism, a craving for love and affection, a considerable sadistic potential, and a blatant disregard for the rules and regulations that govern the life of middle-class society. We started to work on a twice-a-week schedule and, for the next four years, Liz worked very hard. She finished college, and applied to and was accepted into graduate school in psychology. She also became a much more honest and law-abiding citizen. She began to extricate herself from that radical lesbian therapy collective, which was a costly proposition, since she thereby lost a major source of referrals, as well as access to fraudulent insurance reimbursements. Liz took pride in her slow emergence from the untrained, crooked, underground economy that she had been a part of, and she pursued the attempt to "make an honest woman out of herself" with a vengeance. Her social life remained impoverished; she had a few acquaintances, some rather circumscribed relationships with colleagues, no friends, and no romantic life.

Her feelings towards her therapist alternated between utter admiration and, therefore, the impulse to imitate what she thought she saw, and utter denigration and hatred. In the art of provocation Liz was a genius; her rages could be heard out on the street, her foot-stomping, when she was enraged, could be felt on the floor below. She once shredded her new, and what she said was her *only*, winter coat in front of me, with her bare hands, even though it was 10 degrees below freezing during that day. Many times she ran out of a session because she felt misunderstood; she would call at all hours of the night, only to hang up. These rages usually occurred in response to narcissistic injuries, or as a reaction to insufficient praise for accomplishments. Her verbal productions could, at times, be vile, pure gutter language. For example, in response to queries on my part with respect to explanations given about her actions, she would typically shout: "Of course you could not possibly understand this, after all, *you suck cock!*" (meaning, you are heterosexual, you are corrupted as a woman and as a feminist). Liz's hatred for men was indeed bottomless.

During the fourth year of treatment, when she herself became concerned at the intensity of her mood swings, she finally accepted the observation that these swings were extremely cyclical, occurring once every month. She allowed for the possibility that her menstrual cycle and her hormone levels might have something to do with her "nosedives" as she called them, and that she might want to consider medication after all. Since seeing a male physician was entirely out of the question—in fact, the mere suggestion of that possibility was again indicative of my lack of empathy and my degree of corruption by the "male medical establishment"—she consulted her feminist internist, who prescribed a tricyclic antidepressant. At first, her condition seemed to improve, and she had fewer outbursts. But each successive month, their intensity increased. After one particularly powerful flare-up, during which she had barely contained her impulse to destroy me or my office, and at the end of which she again "quit" therapy and had run home, she consented to see my psychopharmacologist, who diagnosed bipolar disorder. He prescribed Lithium, Tegretol, and a small amount of antidepressant. After several months of this new regimen her moods stabilized dramatically. The side effects, however, seemed to interfere with her intellectual functioning.

Unfortunately, pharmacological mood regulation has no bearing whatsoever on character pathology. In fact, as will be shown in Chapter ten, it was one particular aspect of her character structure, the element of psychopathy, which finally undermined her treatment.

Obviously, the severity of a given bipolar disorder is a prime variable in determining how a given patient will fare in life. However, life circumstances, temperament, character armor, also play a major role. William, who combined his outsized appetites with an enormous amount of discipline, as well as charm, was a successful man when he started therapy. His identity was stable and well-defined. The presenting problem was "free-floating anxiety." He could be treated successfully without ever addressing directly the bipolar nature of some of his problems, without his ever needing medication, and by avoiding the term "addiction" altogether. Instead, by focusing on his midlife issues, strengthening his third marriage, finding new and healthier outlets for his energy, such as golf, and by mediating some of the stresses generated by his complicated family system, he slowly lost interest in many of his previous obsessions such as betting, his whores, drugs—though not yet alcohol—and his anxiety has diminished considerably.

Strictly speaking, Karl could have probably easily lived the rest of his life without medication and without those six months of therapy. He would have joined the vast army of vaguely anhedonic people who muddle through life without too many highs or lows. Had he achieved a slightly more comfortable position financially, had his job been just slightly more rewarding, this might well have happened. As it was, life in general, but particularly the prospect of old age in New York under such cramped circumstances, was frightening enough to him to propel him towards further therapeutic help.

Mary, on the other hand, from a certain point on, could not survive without medication, and she will probably need at least some of it for the rest of her life. Additionally, dealing with her social isolation, her low self-esteem, and her fear of people is of equal importance, and it will have a bearing on the *amount* of medication she will need. Providing her with vocational and interpersonal satisfactions will greatly reduce the amount of stress she experiences, and it will help her deal with those stresses that are unavoidable.

Liz, in contrast to the others, never lived a "normal," middle-class life. She truly never knew the rules of the game. Life had always been an extremely tumultuous ordeal. The financial and professional rewards that were not forthcoming from her efforts, she simply wrestled from the system quite literally, by hook or crook. Nothing in her upbringing had provided her with the tools for creating or maintaining intimate and rewarding relationships. Furthermore, an assortment of learning disabilities made her academic pursuits much more difficult than they should have been, given her intelligence. Her at times regal disregard for honesty and for financial obligations has created a complicated network of aliases, lies, denials, and debts that will all have to be addressed and remedied. She has to learn intimate and social skills in order to ease her chronic sense of victimization, frustration, and loneliness. Finally, her grandiosity has to be replaced with a genuine sense of mastery.

CHAPTER THREE

History

How People Conceptualized Mental Illness and Its Treatment

Academic psychology and psychoanalysis are essentially brain-children of the 20th century. Madness, on the other hand, is as old as the human race. Its origins, the causes of mania and depression, have puzzled philosophers, physicians, and theologians throughout history. How people conceptualize mental illness tells us a great deal about how they see themselves. Insanity, after all, is a mirror image—albeit a distorted one—of our hidden self, with all its possibilities. We wonder, what is it that has gone wrong in the melancholic? Is the problem in the mind, the brain, the blood, the bodily organs, or is melancholia due to some supernatural force taking possession of the afflicted person? The answers to these questions have varied over time and from one culture to another.

In the absence of empirical information about the etiology of mood disorders and other forms of mental illness, society needed theories about the subject in order to devise forms of treatment, punishment, even the annihilation of people suffering from madness. The attitudes towards and the understanding of mental illness have ranged from the entirely empirical to the fantastic and from the purely misanthropic to the truly humane. If we look at the various explanatory schemes devised in the course of history, three basic trends can be distinguished: the magical, the organic, and the psychological.

In the history of Western thought, the earliest explanations were theological. In Homeric writings (~1000 BC) people suffering from insanity were thought of as having offended the gods, who then punished them by causing them to act in ways that were crazy. Ulysses, when deranged, plowed sand instead of his fields. Ajax, tortured by delusions, killed sheep instead of his human enemies. When he regained his senses and saw what he had done, he committed suicide. The specific symptoms displayed by a given patient were assumed to indicate which one of the gods had been offended. For example, if the patient uttered a piercing cry, he was thought of as imitating a horse; consequently it probably was Poseidon who had been affronted. Treatment, however, was not punitive in its intent, it was meant to cure. Aesculapian priests, for example, would induce a deep or "incubation" sleep, during which the patient would receive dream inspiration as well as instructions on how to get better.

During the seventh to fifth century BC, Greek philosophy, which at that time was synonymous with science in general, focused almost exclusively on the scientific understanding of the cosmos, on the attempt to build a comprehensive cosmological theory based on materialistic principles: matter, force, and motion. All matter was thought to originate from water. Later, competing schools of thought added air, fire, and earth as the ultimate building blocks of life. The rhythms of life, of the stars, and of life and death were assumed to be interrelated. The four basic elements of the earth (fire, water, air, and the earth itself) were thought to be reflected in the human body as the basic qualities of heat (blood), dryness (phlegm), moisture (yellow bile), and cold (black bile), and were believed to be found in the heart, brain, liver, and spleen, respectively. During the fifth century, the golden age of Greek medicine, madness was looked at as a physical disorder and the term melancholia (*melaina chole,* meaning black bile) was coined. What is called "humoralism"—the notion of bodily humors as crucial elements in health and disease—originated with Empedocles (490–430 BC) and was elaborated by Hippocrates (460–375 BC), known as the father of modern medicine. The elements, responsible for the functioning of the human organism, were thought to be the four humors: blood, yellow bile, black bile, and phlegm. The four humors correspond to the four seasons: spring, summer, autumn, and winter. The four seasons, in turn, correspond to the four basic elements: air, fire, earth, and water. Their principal characteristics are: warm and moist, warm and dry, cold and dry, and cold and moist.

In addition to the humors, the position of the stars was believed to influence human health and illness. For example, people born under the sign of Venus were particularly vulnerable to melancholia because its place in the universe corresponds to the place in the body where the spleen is, and it is the spleen which is the principal producer of black bile. In general, in Greek medicine, mental illness was thought of as a psychological reflection of physiological disturbances. According to Greek medicine, mental and physical health are contingent on a proper balance between the four humors and their respective influence on the brain. Hippocrates claimed that it is the brain—not the heart—which constitutes the most important human organ, since the brain is the interpreter of consciousness. The Greeks recognized the following forms of mental illness: epilepsy, mania, melancholia, and paranoia. The unique contribution made by Greek culture was the emphasis on rationality as opposed to demonology, the assumption that natural phenomena must have natural rather than religious explanations—for example, an excess of black bile leads to melancholia.

That does not mean that religious explanations disappeared; they existed side by side with the rational-empirical approach, but it was the latter that provided the ideas about how the victim of a mental affliction should be treated. Consequently, treatment methods were geared towards alleviating this presumed humoral imbalance: purging, drugs, soothing music, etc. The Greeks even practiced their own form of shock therapy. Patients suffering from catatonic stupor were thrown off a steep cliff and into the ocean where a second physician waited with a boat to fish the patient out of the water. Needless to say, temporarily at least, it worked.

Though the Greeks primarily addressed the pain, and the impairment that is associated with mental illness, they were nevertheless also astutely aware of its positive and creative aspects. Both Socrates (470–399 BC) and Plato (372–287 BC) believed in the concept of "divine madness." According to Plato, no one achieves inspiration and philosophical truth when in his right mind and Socrates claimed that the greatest blessings come by way of madness, madness that is heaven-sent. In contrast to Hippocrates, Plato saw the soul as the governing principle of the body. It consists of the rational soul and the irrational one. Since reason is eternal, God placed it in the skull, in the place nearest to heaven. The irrational soul resides in the rest of the body. The rational soul is the one which governs the organism as a whole. However, the souls freely communicate with each other, and through bodily organs. Galen (131–200 AD), the great Roman atomist, introduced the concept of the four temperaments: sanguine, choleric, melancholic, and phlegmatic. He speculated that some forms of mental illness might also be caused not by an imbalance of humors, but by lesions in the brain. Cicero (106–43 BC), perhaps the first psychologist in Western thought, claimed that instead of humors being the causes of melancholia, it is caused by an excess of strong emotions such as anger, grief, and fear. He was also the first thinker to conceptualize the notion of psychosomatic illness as the product of strong emotions.

During the classical era, surrounding cultures, such as Persia, India, Mesopotamia, and Syria, but particularly Egypt, explained and treated melancholia in ways that were very similar to those of the Greeks. On the whole, the theories of mental illness were medical and empirical in orientation and treatment was uniformly humane. This approach lasted for roughly a thousand years, from 600 BC to 400 AD. With the advent of

Christianity, all that changed drastically. Rationality and humanism in the treatment of the mentally ill mostly disappeared, not to reemerge until the French Revolution, which not accidentally coincided with the last witch-burning in Europe.

During the fourth century, Constantine, seeking the aid of the Christians against his enemies, declared Christianity the official religion of the Roman Empire, thereby forging an allegiance between the church and the state that lasted well over a thousand years. Churches and monasteries became the prime dispensers of medicine, while secular medicine was not only secondary, it was also adjudicated to be in conflict with prevailing doctrines. St. Augustine declared God to be the sole source of healing. Since in his view the writings of classical antiquity represented a source of sexual temptation, he advocated that they be avoided by all good Christians. In general, saving souls superseded the task of treating troubled minds. Psychiatry in the Middle Ages returned to prescientific demonology: treatment became synonymous with penance, coercion, punishment, even exorcism. This shift was due to two intellectual or rather, theological, developments:

1. By the late fourth century the Christian Church had come to use the term "acedia" to designate a constellation of feeling states and behaviors that were considered to be objectionable and unusual and ultimately sinful—namely a sense of dejection, distress, sadness, and immobility, which seemed to affect monks primarily. Similar descriptions of this particular manifestation of depression can be found among the writings of ancient Egyptians, where it was described as an affliction of desert monks, fighting temptations, particularly those which threatened their state of celibacy and solitary life, which among some of them seems to have evoked clinical depression. John Cassian (360–435 AD) also recognized that acedia was particularly common among people living alone and who practiced celibacy. He identified the following symptoms: carelessness, weakness, exhaustion, apathy, anguish, sadness, low spirits, and sloth. Cassian, relying on St. Paul as his authority, prescribed

hard physical labor as a cure, together with the victim's further isolation from his fellow monks.

2. According to the theology of that time, acedia arose not only from forces inside the monk; it could also be caused by demons tempting the ascetic from without. While the Greeks had focused on those aspects of melancholia that interfered with *living*, and therefore recommended joyful activities, including sexual intercourse, as aids to treatment, the early Christians, in contrast, focused on acedia's ability to interfere with the goals of asceticism, namely celibacy and hard work. Consequently, they prescribed isolation and self-flagellation as the proper therapeutic measures. Acedia as an embodiment of evil spirits, even the devil himself, attacked the ascetic to tempt him. In that function it constituted one of the eight principal temptations which later became the seven cardinal sins. Gregory the Great (540–604 AD) reduced the list of cardinal sins from eight to seven by deleting pride. However, since pride was considered the root of *all* sin, its importance was really intensified by the deletion. Though Gregory dropped acedia from the list of sins, he nevertheless retained its equivalent, namely "dejection."

St. Hildegard of Bingen (1098–1179) added an interesting twist to the theories of melancholia by connecting the humor theory of the classical era with the Fall of Man. By eating the apple in paradise, she theorized, Adam developed a melancholic temperament; the melancholic humor was curdling his blood. Melancholia, therefore, was Adam's punishment, to be borne by the entire race as an incurable hereditary evil.

Given the view of depression as a cardinal sin, instead of illness, it should not be surprising that the excessive expression of guilt, typical of the depressive, rather than constituting a universal symptom, is in fact quite unique to the Judeo-Christian world.

St. Thomas of Aquinas (1225–1274) introduced the Aristotelian worldview into medieval thought. However, by subordinating Aristotelian thought to Christian revelation, it became an impediment to scientific inquiry, rather than the stimulus which it had been for the Greeks. St. Thomas declared the separation between body and soul to be absolute in that the soul exists independently of the body. Rational powers are *not* functions of any bodily organs, including those of the brain. Furthermore, with the teachings of St. Thomas, the notion of work as constituting a God-pleasing activity—*"ad majorem Dei gloriam "*—entered Western thought for the first time.

Acedia was still associated primarily with temptation, the perversion of appetites, which included an aversion to spiritual good. Scholastic psychology believed in a system of passions of which *tristitia* and *gaudium* (sorrow and joy) was one opposing pair. *Tristitia* was considered to be the Christian's sensitivity and therefore, response to evil and sin, regardless of the question whether they are real or imaginary, present, past, or future. According to St. Paul, two kinds of *tristitia* have to be distinguished: a positive and a negative one; the positive form leads to penance and salvation, while the other leads to death. The wholesome form of *tristitia* originates in an aversion to and consequently penitence for sins, and a desire for spiritual perfection, while the objectionable form of *tristitia* presumably was caused by worldly preoccupations and distress.

While originally the problems of acedia and *tristitia* had been an object of scrutiny only with respect to the life and spiritual well-being of monks and of the clergy, it was now recognized as an affliction of laypersons as well. Because the fourth Lateran Council in 1215/16 made confession obligatory for everybody, the population as a whole now had to be acquainted with its nature, thereby giving rise to the production of a vast amount of literature on penitence and sin. Now the temptations of the monks had also become one of the cardinal sins of every man, and the general population had to be instructed about what constituted sin and how to recognize its existence. Acedia was described as spiritual idleness or neglect in performing spiritual duties, idleness, and indolence. The standard English term for sin became sloth, and as such it included many worldly aspects, such as neglect of the obligations to one's profession, laziness, inattention, etc. Thomas Aquinas's notion of work as constituting an essential element of man's nature and as God's plan for men, coupled with the description of acedia as dejection and passivity, introduced an entirely new element into the picture; its consequences, however, were not fully evident until after the Reformation—namely, that the sin of acedia means primarily *the simple failure to work*, which may lead to poverty, homelessness, vagrancy, and begging. It seems that notorious institutions such as the infamous Hotel Salpêtrière, which lumped together criminals, the mentally ill, and the poor, goes back to this crucial connection between depression and poverty. Once this equation had been forged, *busyness*, in conjunction with fortitude and spiritual joy, became the principal antidotal virtues to combat acedia in all its forms. Additionally, with the rise of cities in the Middle Ages, urban leaders increasingly faced the problem of growing masses of able-bodied poor, which fit the neglect-idleness-indolence theory of acedia.

During the 13th and 14th centuries, another manifestation of mental turpitude began to dominate the picture, namely witchcraft. Up until then the truly mad had been a community concern and were treated relatively humanely. The theological imperative to pursue witch hunts, originally designed to eliminate or at least to control heretics, now included mental patients who were thought of as possessed by evil demons, or by Satan himself. The odd and the old, and women in all stations of life, became its targets. The Dark Ages were very dark indeed, particularly for the mentally ill, many of whom were probably less deranged than their clerical persecutors. The infamous *Malleus Maleficarum*, published in 1486, is an immense compendium of all the signs and indicators for diabolic possession, relationships with the devil, and all the telltale signs of witchcraft. It unleashed a torrent of persecutions, trials, and burnings for witchcraft, devil worship, and satanic possession as evidenced by the symptoms of mental illness.

Since the origins of mental derangement were thought to be both entirely diabolical in nature and always evil in intent, they constituted sufficient grounds for torture and death. The *Malleus Maleficarum*, probably one of the most inhumane documents ever written, which went through countless revisions over the next 200 years—during Descartes' lifetime alone it went through 16 revisions—resulted in the mutilation, torture, or death of countless innocents—mental patients, adults, and children alike.

While the excesses of the witch hunts eventually ceased, over the next several centuries very little changed in the understanding of and general attitudes towards mental diseases. That does not mean that secular medicine and science did not make valuable and therapeutically useful observations—they did— but several socially powerful forces prevented the integration of these ideas into the official doctrine that governed the actual treatment of mentally ill people. These forces were primarily political and religious. Religion provided the major impediment towards studying the brain. Until Descartes, the psyche and/or human mind, were not seen as legitimate areas of scientific inquiry. As long as St. Thomas's doctrine held fast, the mind of man as God's proudest creation was not to be questioned and his immortal soul was not to be analyzed or dissected. God's powerful counterpart, the devil, is forever busy trying to snatch souls away from God, thus interfering with God's plans by taking possession of his proudest achievement. Man's only role in all of this, his only hope in this scheme, is to strive for forgiveness, to contain and combat evil wherever it raises its ugly head, which is just about everywhere. This was particularly true because the definition of evil or of sin as by no means a purely religious or spiritual one. It was in many respects synonymous with social deviance and it included any deed and any population that did not fit into the rigid class structure and its corresponding rules and regulations which covered all aspects of everyday life, no matter how minute. Thus the oppression was twofold. It was aimed at maintaining a religious belief system and a social class system simultaneously. Poverty—though not vagrancy—had been acceptable during the Middle Ages because it was accepted as part of God's will, and charity, therefore, constituted a Christian duty. The poor, the homeless, the unemployed, and the mentally ill were cared for in some fashion in the communities where they lived. However, as the population expanded and as the cities increasingly became the repositories for ever-increasing numbers of the poor, the homeless, and the unemployed, the mentally ill were lumped together with other indigenous groups, declared a threat to law and order, and were incarcerated, often in the same institutions, the most famous of which were the Hotel Salpêtrière in Paris and Bedlam in London. Since mental illness was seen as, among other things, sloth, it was a sin, and therefore had to be punished and contained. Patients were shackled and chained, kept in dungeons, and put on ships that were then abandoned. In many medieval towns they were put in the *Tollhaus* (asylum) or were given a flogging, some clothes and money, and were chased out of town and told never to return. However, the treatment of mental patients during the Middle Ages was still benign compared with that administered during the 16th and 17th centuries. For example, for almost two centuries the St. Elizabeth Hospital in England had been a genuine asylum, a relatively benign institution, before it became known as Bedlam. During the 18th century it became a famous Sunday excursion place for the good citizens of London who came to watch and to torture mad men and women through the iron gates and fences that contained them. In fact, during that period, given the choice between an asylum and jail, jail was usually the better deal for the inmate. While sanitary conditions were the same in both places, prisoners at least did not have to endure the same insults to their bodies, such as bloodletting, purging emetics, and so-called harmless tortures.

Obviously, the church did not provide the *only* theories about the etiology and treatment of mental and physical illness. Some of the writings of antiquity survived, and they served secular medicine. During the Renaissance many of the Greek texts, translated by Arab scholars, reached Europe. Thus the religious and the secular theories, the supernatural and the empirical, existed side by side and sometimes even within the same person. Kepler, for example, was as much of an astrologer as he was an astronomer. Physicians and artists during that period belonged to the same guilds, with anatomy constituting a common concern. Leonardo da Vinci (1452–1519) was both anatomist and artist.

The philosophers of the Enlightenment, starting with Francis Bacon and including writers such as Claude Helvetius, Baron d'Holbach, Condillac, and Destutt de Tracy, made human irrationality one of the major foci of their inquiries. Bacon's (1626) famous "idols" (of the tribe, den, marketplace, and theater) "are the deepest fallacies of the human mind; they do not deceive in particulars as the rest, by clouding and ensnaring judgement; but from corrupt predisposition, or bad complexion of the mind, which distorts and infects all the anticipations of the understanding. For the mind darkened by the covering of the body, is far from being a flat, equal and clear mirror that receives and reflects the rays without mixture, but rather a magical glass full of superstitions and apparitions." (p. 239)

While Bacon excluded the church and the state from his considerations, the other thinkers did not, and their writings were printed mostly abroad and distributed secretly through a quite extensive network of underground publishers and distribution chains.

Robert Burton's *Anatomy of Melancholy,* published in 1621, constitutes probably the largest compendium on the subject that has ever been assembled by a nonphysician. It is also a prime example of the parallelism of the different modes of thinking. With respect to the causes of melancholy, Burton lists the following: God, the devil, witches, stars, humors, physical illness, poverty, food, vehement desires—in other words, any and all causes originating in the divine, physiological, social, physiological, astrological, and other spheres. Venus and hot baths are equally important as causal agents, and his therapeutic recommendations varied accordingly.

While in the course of the 16th and 17th centuries humor

theory was superseded first by chemical explanations—spirits, sulphur, water, and earth and its derivatives in the bloodstream, with the spleen in the role of fermenter—the 18th century shifted to a more mechanical explanation, namely that mental disorders resulted from the hydrodynamics of the blood and that in turn affected the flow of animal spirits in the nervous system, and thus caused disordered thoughts, even delirium. Theorists such as Pitcairn (1642–1727) did not discard the humor theory as a whole, but they focused on the circulation of humors rather than on their relative distribution. After all, this being the age of Newton, physicians were quite inclined to see the human body as a hydraulic machine.

Psychiatry as a medical-empirical science could not become an established discipline as long as Aquinas's doctrine of the separation between body and soul was the only ruling doctrine. Spinoza originated the concept of psychophysiological parallelism, which states that mind and body are inseparable because they are identical; the human organism experiences its bodily processes psychologically as affects, thoughts, and desires. Psychology and physiology are two aspects of the same entity: the living organism. However, Spinoza, who wrote these theories in opposition to Descartes (1596–1650), was declared a heretic and was promptly excommunicated from his synagogue. Had he not lived in liberal Holland, he might well have been burned at the stake.

Descartes' theories pertaining to the laws governing body and mind were the concepts that were to prevail simply because they did not put medicine in conflict with theology: the mind and the soul exist independently of each other and they are governed by different sets of laws and principles. All material things are divisible; the mind and the soul are not (the indivisibility argument); therefore they are qualitatively different from the material world. Mind and soul are created by God and they are immortal. They are governed by nonmechanistic and immaterial principles. The human body, in contrast, together with all plants and animals, obeys the law of physics which are

God-given and universal. Life is physics; the human body itself is a machine.

Hence, qualities such as perceptions, will, pleasure, and pain do not reside in matter; they exist only in the immaterial realm, the human mind. The human brain itself can be of no use to pure understanding. Cartesian Dualism became the theoretical basis on which medicine and theology could begin to go their separate ways. With the soul remaining the province of theology, the body, including the brain, now became the subject of medicine, which in the 18th century finally dislodged demons from the etiology of human illness. This period was also the age of the great systematizers and of important social reform movements. What Linnaeus (1707–1778) did for plant life, early psychiatry did for mental illness. Particularly in France, nosology became a central focus.

The systematic observations of patients allowed for the discovery of clusters of symptoms and a more precise knowledge of the probable causes of a given disorder. In France this work was done primarily by Pinel (1745–1826) and his contemporaries, Esquirol, Falret, Baillarget. In Germany in the 19th century the work was continued by Kraeplin and Bleuler and in the U.S. by Adolf Meyer. At the end of the 19th century, depression, manic-depressive insanity, as it was called, and schizophrenia (dementia praecox) were established as distinct clinical entities, each with specific features and different prognoses. In terms of social reform two names stand out: Pestalozzi, for the humane education of children, and Philippe Pinel for the liberation of mental patients. When Pinel first took the chains off the patients at the Hotel Salpêtrière and substituted decent food, air, sanitation, and medical treatment in 1795, six years after the storming of the Bastille, he was considered to be as mad as his patients. He persisted, and gradually the other asylums followed suit.

However, this era of enlightenment and rationality was also a period of outstanding successes of famous quacks: phrenologists, homeopathists, and Mesmer's animal magnetism were equally popular. While the French Revolution—"the triumph of reason"—took place, the last witch in Europe was burned.

Soon the triumph of reason and empiricism gave way to profound disillusionment with the power of reason. A romantic reaction in the form of a rediscovery of the soul and the irrational, the appreciation of the depth of the human psyche and instinct and passions became the focal points of interest. Man's struggle with his internal self became more fascinating than his struggle with the external world. *Weltschmerz* and mysticism in the humanities, and a return to absolutist principles in government, and a religious resurgence all characterized the period from 1789 to 1840. Yet it also gave birth to scientists of such importance as Charles Darwin in biology, Hermann von Helmholz in psychology, and Rudolf von Virchow and Louis Pasteur in medicine. Nerve impulses and cell biology were discovered and neurology was in its early stages.

By the end of the century, medicine had made remarkable progress in diagnosing the causes of a large number of specific diseases. Many of the traditional scourges of mankind were discovered not to be the will of God, a punishment for sin, but simply the work of bacteria that could be counteracted by better sanitation and specific medications. It seemed quite logical to assume that mental illnesses had similar pathogenic causes and that they could be treated similarly. It seemed only a matter of understanding what physiologically happens in the brain of the mentally ill, in order to cure it. After all, by discovering the spirochete that causes syphilis, and eventually dementia, one particular form of psychosis (tertiary syphilis affecting the brain) was now understood, though not yet cured. While general medicine progressed, none of the aspirations of psychiatry for simple medical cures had materialized by the time the century ended.

In order to understand the history of psychiatry, psychology, and psychoanalysis in the 20th century it is important to understand the philosophical underpinnings of the various life sciences at that time. For the most part, psychiatry as a branch of medicine then restricted its inquiry to two areas: mental *illness* and its organic causes, including genetics.

The industrial revolution and corresponding urbanization had meanwhile created what, among other things, became known as the "Social Problem": a large proletariat, vast unemployment, alcoholism, crime, juvenile delinquency, and all the medical, social, and mental pathologies that are the result of poverty, child labor, and malnutrition. These problems could no longer be contained by outright repression, appeased by paternalistic welfare reforms, or understood merely in terms of immorality, stupidity, perversity, or constitutional depravity on the part of its victims. Though as explanatory concepts they have not altogether vanished, even to this day, all of these phenomena and the political imperative of finding an effective remedy nevertheless gave rise to psychology, educational psychology, sociology, and a host of related disciplines (Schad, 1972). Some of the most impressive investigations into the causes of juvenile delinquency were made by legal scholars and by psychiatrists and social workers. As was the case with the psychiatry of that time, the emphasis was on the phenomenology of the pathology, the size of the problem; to count and to classify was the first order of the day. The main emphasis was on psychopathology, rather than on the mind in general, which was still mainly the province of philosophy. Besides, the identification and the classification of pathogenic elements in the human environment provided enough of a challenge for the social sciences for decades to come.

In European philosophy, the legacy of German romanticism was still a powerful influence. Its emphasis on the mind as pure abstraction and the notion of a world spirit (*Weltgeist*) as *the* force in history, an entity which aims at coming into its own with human beings and human history as its mere vehicle, a notion which is immensely appealing and convincing, attributes social change to the "cunning of reason" and, therefore, has no use for any individual psychology. History, according to Hegel, is the history of the progress in the consciousness of freedom.

Likewise, Marx's historical materialism conceptualizes man as essentially a victim of economic and historical forces, rather than as a psychological being in which individual history, social forces, and biological imperative interact and are in turn reshaped. Put differently, at the beginning of this century, in terms of laying the foundations for a unified theory of human motivation, the field was—at least theoretically—wide open. However, given the division of labor between the life sciences, the social and political demands made on them, and the biological and medical knowledge of that time, and finally, the accident that Sigmund Freud's genius came to dominate the field of psychotherapy, it is quite understandable that it took almost another 80 years for such a theory to emerge and to establish itself.

While historically the Cartesian mind-body dualism had, among other things, provided the basis for a medical approach to mental illness and, consequently, for a more humane treatment for its victims, it also posed an intellectual obstacle to an understanding of man as the only creature who, as Ernest Becker (1965) put it, "is a body and has a body." We are the only animals who can use a part of their bodies, namely the brain, to contemplate itself. Unless one conceives of the mind either as a spiritual force that cannot be located in human physiology or as the doings of a physical entity, the intellectual challenge is to transcend this split, an intellectual feat we are just now beginning to accomplish.

Freud, along with his contemporaries the psychiatrist Adolf Meyer and the philosopher John Dewey and psychologist William James, had been quite aware of this problem. Adolf Meyer, who already used the term psychobiology in 1915, attempted to integrate the various social, biological, and psychological forces that interact in any given individual, and to chart these influences over the course of a life span. His focus, in contrast to that of his colleagues in Europe, was on the adaptive capacities of the human organism, rather than on the nosology of psychopathology. Meyer viewed mental illness as a faulty adaptation, one that was due to a whole variety of pathogenic influences impinging over time. His "life charts," tracing these stress factors, come quite close to the contemporary concept of a "final common pathway." William James, in his Principles of General Psychology (1890), made an attempt to integrate the sense organs and the brain with human behavior and motivation. However, his understanding of the connection between sensations and emotions, which became known as the James-Lange theory of emotions, made the organs of sense perception the starting point, and the expression of emotion the link between perception and feelings. According to James we are sad because we cry, not the other way around. Nevertheless, his and John Dewey's psychology of human motivation which focuses on man as primarily a symbolic and a social animal, one in which symbolic motivations outweigh organismic ones, is better suited for a psychobiology of emotions than the Freudian model of man as motivated by biological drives and instincts. However, their influence on psychoanalysis and psychiatry remained negligible until Ernest Becker incorporated their ideas into his transactional models of depression and schizophrenia.

Freud, who had been trained as a neurologist, shared the scientific optimism of his time, the hope that a general psychology could be rooted in neurology and that mental ills could be understood medically. However, at the time he wrote "On Aphasia" (1891) and "The Project for a Scientific Psychology" (1895) the knowledge of both the structure and the function of the brain were still too primitive to make this possible. It is remarkable, though, that between the neurological facts that had been established and Freud's intuition, he was surprisingly accurate when he postulated in "The Project" that there are pathways of energy, that their usage over time established learning, memory, fixation, and cathexes. He also presumed that it took specific levels of energy for the neurons to fire across the synapse between the neurons, that accumulation of energy produced discomfort (*Unlust*) and the need to redistribute energy in different directions or pathways. By the time he wrote his *General Outline of Psychoanalysis* (1905), however, Freud concluded sadly: "We know two things about what we call our psyche (or mental life): firstly, its bodily organ and scene of action, the brain (or nervous system) and, on the other hand, our acts of consciousness, which are immediate data and cannot be further explained by any sort of description. Everything that lies in between is unknown to us, and the data do not include any direct relation between those two terminal points of our knowledge" (1949, p. 1). This, essentially, remained the definitive statement on the subject for the rest of Freud's life, and there is no evidence that he tried to incorporate the neurology of the 20th century into his psychoanalytic theories.

Assuming that psychology had to explain biologically what makes organisms move, Freud settled on the metaphorical concepts of drives or instincts, which do not correspond to any real biological entities. Unlike Dewey and James, who looked to man's symbol world to explain the force and the direction of human action, Freud looked for the physical engine, the source of power in the physiology of man. It did not occur to him that organisms move and that there is no need to search for a why— that it is inherent in the concept of life. Living means moving. His hypothetical concept of drive or instinct implies a type of power as well as a direction or goal. The "death instinct" assumes that all living organisms strive to return to an inorganic state. In his model, man resembles a hydraulic engine which operates with a fixed amount of energy—very much like the steam in a locomotive—and this force can be directed, rerouted, attach itself to specific objects, and can be turned back upon itself. Instinctual goals and the demands of civilized life are basically in conflict; civilization is bought at the price of neurosis. Additionally, the drives and the components of the psyche are in conflict with each other—intrapsychic conflict.

Having concluded that what was known about the brain and the central nervous system did not provide us with enough knowledge for the understanding of human motivation, Freud focused increasingly on function rather than structure. The structural components of the mind are meant to be metaphorical; they pertain to the psyche rather than the brain. They are the ego, the superego, and the id, and the conscious, the unconscious, and the preconscious.

In the psychoanalytic model, depression has two principal sources: anger turned upon the self and object loss (melancholia). In the case of melancholia the lost love object is taken into the ego, which means that the self-reproaches, typical of the melancholic, are really statements about the love object who abandoned the melancholic. If the relationship to a love object is an ambivalent one, the aggressive component cannot be expressed for fear of losing the object altogether, a loss which the dependent part of a dyad cannot risk. The psyche, then, without help from the outside, transducts one affect—aggression—into another, namely depression. Freud himself did not have a very convincing theory of the causes of mania. He proposed that an excess of libido or aggression threatens to flood the ego. Mania defends against this danger. But essentially mania cannot really be explained by psychoanalysis, and leading psychoanalysts, such as Edith Jacobson, have all along proposed that mania, besides being a manifestation of superego pathology, is also the result of endogenous and as yet unknown physiological processes. In terms of metapsychology, the model of the mind that is employed here to explain psychological phenomena, the Freudian model, is quite similar to the working of what then was the most advanced technology, namely the steam engine, and it corresponds to the predominant theoretic model in physics at that time, namely the exchange of particles. The same is true today: the model of the mind in current thinking in many respects resembles, and yet transcends, that of the computer with the notion of "information processing and transmission" as its basic underlying concept. What distinguishes the mind from the computer is the computer's capacity to conceive of many possibilities simultaneously. While the mind is aware of all these possibilities, the body/brain expresses only one particularity as it were. In that sense, the mind/body relationship has been compared to the wave/particle duality of light as conceptualized in Heisenberg's uncertainty principle and quantified by quantum mechanics (Zohar, 1990).

While psychoanalysis has been by no means the only model of the mind, it certainly has until recently been the dominant one used by psychotherapists. Consequently the different life sciences have run on parallel tracks with not too much corrective interaction, a development that probably would have saddened Freud immensely. Freud had had no choice but to create hypothetical constructs to explain psychic phenomena. Not enough was known about the physiology of the brain to prove or disprove his metatheory. Besides, psychoanalysis or psychoanalytic psychotherapy, compared to other forms of treatment for mental disorders, proved to be singularly effective for the treatment of milder disorders, which explains at least in part why Freudian and neo-Freudian theory predominated in the field of psychotherapy for as long as they have. Freud, from the beginning, restricted the applicability of psychoanalysis to the neuroses, disorders which by the diagnostic standards of today include many types of psychopathology, ranging from neurosis to borderline pathology, but exclude schizophrenia and the major psychoses.

The very concept "mental illness" encapsulates all the conceptual problems inherent in the phenomenon. "Illness" suggests a physiological dysfunction, strictly a challenge for science and scientific therapy. "Mental" gets us into the slippery world of nonscientific, nonempirical, and elusive phenomena that can be observed but cannot as readily be dissected and analyzed by scientific methods. To fully appreciate the intellectual challenge posed by the existence of mania and depression, we first have to look at man both as a social and as a symbolic animal. Additionally, we have to examine some of the most recent findings in basic clinical neuroscience.

CHAPTER FOUR

Psyche

Our Symbolic Universe

While mood disorders are not the exclusive property of humans, madness is. Animals can be driven crazy in the laboratory, but it is not a condition that occurs in the wild. Madness involves cognitive disturbances—confusion about the meaning of symbols—and that is, for the most part, a uniquely human ability. While we share with the nonhuman primates the potential for depression—and possibly mania—the causes are usually vastly more complex because man is primarily a symbolic and a social animal. What makes us vulnerable to madness, as well as to greatness, renders us capable of committing suicide and of composing symphonies, is the fact that we do not have a species-specific environment, one in which the biological blueprint determines its actualization, meanings, motives, or mood regulation.

The human animal is born several years prematurely, a fact which has many far-reaching consequences. It gave the brain, particularly the cortex—the thinking part of the brain—additional time to grow. The dependency of the immature human organism on a primary caretaker means that the young develop attachments of a much more profound nature, which constitutes a blessing and a curse. Attachment means that learning is primarily social learning but, more important, the price of object love is the danger of object loss and corresponding grief. To the extent that we love others, we have to fear that they may die or that they may leave us.

In humans the evolutionary change from a biyearly sexual cycle to continuous sexual receptivity means that the female remains erotic and sexually receptive while rearing children. As a result, we have increasingly complicated social interactions that need to be regulated to take account of the different roles. Without an incest taboo, there would be a jumble of social statuses, instead of a hierarchy based on generational successions. Shared food acquisition requires joint explorations of the environment, shared problem solving, and that means that social life has to be regulated by means other than brute force.

Symbols, language, and abstractions increasingly provided motives and social power until we evolved into an animal which is fully capable of divorcing its symbol world from its biological base.

A species-specific environment is one in which "reality" is nothing other than a reflection of biology. There is a distinct dog world, fly world, snake world, and these worlds are unique to these classes of animals. A frog's brain divides the entire universe only into two classes of objects: bugs and nonbugs. In a species-specific environment the existence of phenomena, be they physical objects, other animals, sounds, smells, or sights, are contingent on the structure of the sense organs of the particular species in question, and the relevance of these phenomena for the animal's survival. A soup bone has a very distinct smell, and therefore meaning for the dog: it will grab it and consume it in the utmost privacy and as quickly as possible. From a visual-aesthetic point of view, the bone has no meaning for the dog whatsoever. The fly, too, will sense the bone as a foodstuff, but the bone itself is not perceived as an object. For the snake, the bone does not exist as a distinct entity at all, it is merely background. The same is true for the Empire State Building: it represents, at best, an object to occupy when the fly wants to rest; it is not distinguished from any other stonelike surface.

Human reality, of course is also limited by our organs of sense perception and by our technological ingenuity. Therefore it is most probable that there are vast numbers of phenomena on this globe that we know nothing about simply because we have no organs to perceive them with and no technology to look for them or measure them. In fact, if I understand some of the basic tenets of modern physics correctly, 90% of the universe is "black matter," which means that we do not have the slightest idea of what 90% of the universe is made of. Atomic particles were not "real" until the 20th century, when technology made them a reality. However, within these biological limitations we essentially "make" our reality what we want or need it to be. It is socially constructed rather than dictated or even suggested by biology.

Our biology tells us very little. We must eat, drink, sleep and procreate. It does not tell us what, where, with whom, or how often. We had to make it up as we went along, which means that most objects around us have no intrinsic or objective reality. They are what we define them as; they are what we attribute to them. Thus the famous evocation, "You must remember this, a kiss is still a kiss," is true only in the movies. Eskimos would be unable to make any sense out of it because kissing to them seems merely silly and unsanitary.

Attributions can and habitually do override biology. For example, Clyde Kluckhohn told the story of the anthropologists who were doing fieldwork with Eskimos and regularly enjoyed a native lunch meat that seemed to be a cross between chicken and tuna and they found it to be extremely tasty. When they discovered, to their utter surprise, that for months on end they had been eating rattlesnake, their stomachs, being ruled by what Kluckhohn calls "the cultural web," protested, and they promptly vomited just thinking about it. Humans will eat poisonous mushrooms; animals know better. We have to learn that in the West the *Amanita muscaria*, perhaps one of the prettiest of the wild mushrooms, can be deadly, even though visually it looks as tempting as a ripe apple. The information that rattlesnakes are nutritious—once they are dead—and that in America *Amanita muscaria* is poisonous (though in other parts of the world it is merely hallucinogenic and therefore precious), is abstract and acquired knowledge and therefore subject to change. It may even vanish entirely and become extinct. For example, in certain parts of Russia, *Amanita muscaria* was so valued for its hallucinogenic properties that some groups of men regularly overcame their revulsion towards drinking human urine to obtain it. Since a large proportion of the active toxin of the *Amanita* is excreted through the urine, one mushroom could be shared by an entire group of hunters, who would then form what must be thought of as a kind of hallucinogenic daisy chain, by passing the urine of the man who first ate the mushroom onto the next, who passed it on to the third, until the toxin was completely used up.

Biologically, what we bring to this world is an action potential, but its realization has to be acquired by each individual and group. Reality, then, is built, invented, reinvented, and negotiated. For purposeful action to be possible, for the organism to move forward, the world around us must be intelligible, and therefore predictable. Without a certain amount of security in the predictability of specific properties of the objects around us, we would be paralyzed by anxiety. I have to be able to trust that the laws of gravity are operating in order to risk stepping out of bed, and I have to be certain that a green traffic light means "walk," in order to cross the street. Prior to the invention of the lightning rod, we could only tolerate the threat represented by thunder and lightning if we could believe that there was a god called Thor, who threw his hammer around when he was angered, but who could be pacified by certain rituals and sacrifices. Furthermore, we also have a limited tolerance for what is called "cognitive dissonance," a fact which a popular television series called *Candid Camera* used to comic advantage. They would show the proverbial sweet little old lady in an affluent suburb who politely asked the cop on the beat where she could buy explosives. The policeman, caught between two contradictory cognitive sets or social clues would be unable to act. All he knew how to do was stare. Sweetness and a request for explosives do not go together.

For individuals and societies, life is only possible if they can answer what John Dewey (1922) has called the four common human questions: (1) What kinds of reactions can I expect from the human objects I encounter? (2) What is the extent, support, and limitation of my power? (3) In what sequence or sequential schema must my actions and my life be embedded? and (4) How can I best orient my actions towards safety and to maximum satisfaction? As humans we are born into a ready-made world of meanings and symbols; in other words, we are born into a pre-existing social reality, a universe of meanings which we experience as "objective reality." The reality which is comprised of the sum total of what "everybody knows" is what Berger and Luckmann (1967) have called "the reality of everyday life." It is there and it is self-evident. How did it get there? Obviously, even the simplest human interaction requires agreed-upon typifications or roles. If nothing else, males and females in the cave knew what to expect of each other in sexual intercourse. Male is he who penetrates. Penetrators are men. Babymakers are women. Human activity, or "externalization," results in social products called social institutions, as well as in physical products, the means of survival.

All human activity is subject to habitualization because habitualization frees the actors from "all those decisions." In that way it is economical in that it saves energy for deliberation and innovation. Furthermore, it makes behavior predictable to those around us. The "here I go again" becomes "here he or she goes again." There may be umpteen ways to get hold of animal flesh. However, a sharpened stick proved one day to be effective. Repetition then transformed all sharpened sticks into what became known, first to the individual and then to the group, as a whole, as "spears." Those who carry spears and who successfully puncture woolly mammoths and who bring back meat become known as hunters, a social role equally understood by actor and spectator alike. Hunting becomes a social institution with its traditions: "Ever since the great hunt, right after the earthquake, we perform a rain dance. We hunt whenever the moon is full," and folklore and legitimations: "The brain of the mammoth gives strength. . . . the most successful hunter makes the best husband," and children born into a clan which discovered hunting experience the reality of the hunt and all it entails as a God-given reality, one which has always existed ("everybody knows that"), and also as a possible script for their own lives. A social role, then, is a vocabulary of motives which orchestrates and implements performance. Roles are an important prerequisite for social interaction. Their relative complementarity or their dissonance determines the relative amounts of conflict or social equilibrium within a given pair or group. Chiefs need Indians, and vice versa. Individuals who are ignorant of or deviant from the existing roles and institutions are considered to be stupid, mentally ill, or depraved. An adult, for example, who enters a college classroom walking on his head can be any of those three things. Depending on the designation, society will instruct, punish, cure, or reform the deviant.

Social roles are only a part of our identity, they constitute one aspect of our social self. In some instances the social self can become our core self. For example, Ernest Becker (1967) has argued that for some of the brokers caught in the stock-market crash of 1929, money and the power to manipulate, control, and generate it, had taken the place of the core self. Consequently, the act of jumping out of a window was merely the physical duplication of a death that had already occurred. However, for most of us, the self-system is a much more complex entity, which comprises a number of different social roles, such as parent, breadwinner, voter, and taxpayer, together with a private self, and supported by varying degrees of self-esteem. In the eyes of the world we may be a lowly bookkeeper; in the eyes of our children we often are God; in the eyes of our spouse we may be a great beauty; and as far as the dog is concerned the hand that pours the puppy chow rules the world. In our private world we may be anything from a great poet to a common criminal. Psychological equilibrium is contingent on a balance and the compatibility of these different parts of the self-system.

Since learning—the acquisition of a universe of meaning and motives—is a social process, originally the product of an interaction between a helpless infant and its caretakers, our sense of reality and our sense of self are extremely vulnerable. Meanings cannot be imparted just symbolically, they must be lived, exercised, confirmed, and experienced as secure parts of our inner world. An object consisting of two planes and four sticks is only a meaningful object recognized reliably as a chair when one has sat on it time and again. Becoming the great baker of mud pies also requires countless repetitions. On the other hand, we also need the time and space to contemplate and reflect on all sittable objects as part of the furniture, on all substances that can make mudpies, and on all the different uses of mud. In other words, we need both: doing and contemplating ("undergoing," as Dewey called it). Since we always operate in two worlds, the object world and the symbol world, we need one to support the other. If they drift apart, we are in trouble, we "lose contact with reality," we are considered to be psychotic.

Even our own bodies are not immune from this process. The bed-wetting child who is told every time it happens that "my Johnny could not possibly do such a thing," must divorce his body from its symbolic representation. Similarly, the anorectic's body, which is in the process of starving to death, does not succeed in notifying the mind that it is anything *but* grossly fat. Even of greater importance in acquiring a sound sense of self and of the reality around us, is the affirmation of it on the part of our significant others. The genius of the mud-pie production needs another, preferably all important, adult in his or her environment who will confirm that the product is indeed a mud pie and that its creation produces pleasure in the eyes of those who see it, and furthermore that it is a great example of its kind. To paraphrase Winnicott (1965): Before we ever see a mirror we see our mother's eyes. What we see in them, throughout our childhood, determines to a very large extent how we see ourselves. The initial reflection of a monstrous infant is one which nobody could ever fully forget. The mud pie that is adjudicated as just some goddamn piece of dirt, useless "schmutz" brought into the house will become just that, and instead of motivating the organism it will inhibit it and with it a piece of curiosity and creativity.

Our vulnerability to the responses of significant others can literally make the difference between life and death. The only empirical study that I know of which investigated the causes of a suicide epidemic in a mental hospital (Kobler & Stotland, 1964) showed that given identical diagnoses, identical degrees of depression, and psychiatric history, the single most important cause of this particular rash of suicides was the loss of self-confidence *on the part of the staff,* which resulted in the fact that they suddenly took unusual suicide precautions. These changes in psychiatric protocol communicated to the patients the fact that the staff no longer had the confidence that they could adequately help their charges. If, in addition, the families of these patients also declared the situation to be hopeless, those patients could no longer fend off despair. To retain hope without seeing it reflected in the environment was too overwhelming a task for these individuals whose problem had been hopelessness to begin with. Once that institution regained its self-concept of being in the forefront of psychiatric knowledge, and as soon as they were able to impart that attitude to their patients, the suicide epidemic ended as quickly as it had begun.

The fact that in humans symbolic rewards outweigh organismic ones, that we can make reality what we want it to be, also accounts for our almost infinite capacity to deal with adversity by making something out of nothing. For example, a broken glass or a bottle are generally regarded as garbage. Much of this kind of garbage has ended up in the oceans. After some time of being tossed about it gets washed ashore, by which time it is opaque and has lost all its sharp edges. To all intents and purposes, *objectively* it is still garbage, and everybody saw it as such until some unknown and ingenious individual named it sea glass, which is collected and exhibited in tall glass jars filled with water and stood on windowsills where the sun illuminates it. To a serious collector a piece of *red* sea glass is worth its weight in gold. This redefinition of garbage has given the old Noxema and Maalox bottles which account for most of the cobalt-blue pieces an entirely new and unanticipated life. No dog in its right mind would ever be interested in catnip as a substitute for rawhide; only humans can reframe garbage into valued treasures and can thereby experience it as a substitute for losses in the stock market. This ability to manipulate reality constitutes one of the most important parts of our coping skills which enable us to withstand stresses that other animals under similar conditions could not withstand as readily as we can. In fact, in terms of unhappiness and depression, there seems to be little or no correlation between the objective reality and the degree of human happiness.

Ever since Durkheim's (1897) classic study of suicide, we know that under the most adverse conditions as, for example, war, suicide rates are at an all-time low. In the population Durkheim studied, age and religion were better predictors for suicide than income or physical health. The fact that wars act as deterrents to suicide is explained by the importance of social cohesion that results when an entire society rallies against a common enemy. Once the war is over, and people return to their private lives, suicide rates go back up to their prewar levels. What, then, if not objective misery, depresses humans as a group? Among other factors, it is the discrepancy between how things are and how things are supposed to be. Robert Merton (1962), in his study of anomie, pointed out that American society which subscribes to the Horatio Alger myth which implies that any person who tries hard enough could, if not be president, at least rise from rags to riches, poses a peculiar problem for most of its citizens. Since the Horatio Alger myth is precisely that—a myth—most people, by the time they have reached middle age, have to account for their inability to achieve that goal. As Merton hypothesized—and as subsequent research has borne out—people are more likely to blame themselves than society and the people who sold them this particular bill of goods.

In a similar vein, recently there has been a wave of articles suggesting that the 1980s notion of "having it all" has similarly depressing results. A society that promotes an ideology which in terms of social rewards such as money and social power keeps upping the ante without offering corresponding opportunities to achieve these goals, is bound to generate depression and low self-esteem. There seems to be a direct correlation between, on the one hand, the emphasis on individualism, personal achievement, the "me first" syndrome, or what Christopher Lash (1976) has called the "culture of narcissism," and on the other, the waning of community concerns and involvement and the incidence of clinical depression. Two recent studies (Buie, 1988) sponsored by the Alcohol, Drug Abuse and Mental Health Administration, found evidence that people born after 1945 are 10 times more likely to suffer from clinical depression than people born during the previous 50 years. The key variables here seem to be the degree to which people feel helpless, hopeless, and lonely, and the extent to which a society offers ideational, familial, or religious buffers to cope with these feelings. The way we construct and interpret the reality we encounter and the way we feel about it are not necessarily the same thing. The mind, defined here as our total field of meanings, has to be distinguished from mood or affect in both manifestation and genesis. Mood regulation, the ability to recover from trauma, the capacity to maintain an expectable degree of happiness, is also socially acquired. It evolves from the interaction between the infant and its primary caretaker. Being properly and consistently soothed and comforted, the infant eventually internalizes the soothing administered by the parent and learns to soothe and calm itself. For this process to succeed, caretaker and child have to be attuned. Mother has to know what is needed and how to be comforting without being intrusive. A child who has been given this initial charge, the skills for the regulation of mood as well as self-esteem, and who has learned to rely on social support systems, has an infinitely greater chance to weather individual disappointments later in life than a child who has not.

Having portrayed the human animal as primarily a symbolic and social one raises a number of intriguing philosophical questions. To start with the most fundamental one: What, then, if anything, is "human nature"? Is man infinitely malleable? Are we "by nature" born good or bad? I cannot offhand think of a single subject that is as likely to start an intellectual battle among behavioral scientists than the validity of Freud's contention that there is such a thing as "primary aggression," a force or instinct that aims to fight and destroy. Put differently, what is the role of biology in human affairs, or, to use Konner's (1982) elegant formulation, what are the constraints on the human spirit? Before addressing this question in the next chapter, it is necessary to return to the conundrum posed by the last section of the previous chapter, namely how do we best conceptualize the phenomena of mental health and mental illness?

The fact that man lacks a species-specific environment obviously does not mean that we are born as psychological putty with no emotional or intellectual inclinations, predispositions, or limitations. After all, we are, like all other living things on this globe, the product of evolution. What we bring to this world is an action potential, a biological blueprint that requires specific environments to unfold. Freud conceived of it as the tension between eros and thanatos, life and death, and since his time there have been quite a few competing schools of thought to explain the nature of that potential. The line of reasoning or inquiry that has empirically withstood the test of time are Bowlby's (1969, 1973, 1988) ground-breaking work on attachment, separation, and loss, Spitz's (1958, 1965) observations of neglected infants, Harlow's (1958, 1971) experiments with monkeys, and all the research that followed from their basic premise, namely, that attachment behavior is the primary behavioral system of the newborn infant. It is born with all other behavioral systems in place, waiting to unfold in a predictable developmental sequence, given a good-enough environment. As mentioned in the introduction, legend has it that King Frederick Barbarossa, in an attempt to find out what language humans would speak if they were not taught a particular language as children, assembled 100 newborn infants. He instructed the nurses who were in charge of raising them to tend to their biological needs *only,* to feed and to change them. They were not to be spoken to or played with, or given any form of psychological sustenance.

Not one of those babies survived the first year. Whether this account is anecdotal or factual does not really matter since Spitz's observations of children left in hospitals and orphanages more than confirm that in the absence of talking, cooing, stroking, in other words, all the interpersonal acts that constitute "mothering," infants can die from miasma (a pathological wasting of tissue not due to malnutrition), fail to thrive, and will develop a wide variety of physiological and psychological disturbances. Harlow and his co-workers observed that monkeys who had had only artificial surrogate mothers to cling to in infancy grew into youngsters unable to relate to their peers and into adults unable to mate, or, if they did, to raise their young. All the empirical evidence we have on humans raised in similar conditions point in the same direction. Human infants are born with a set of perceptumotor mechanisms designed to elicit mothering behavior. If it succeeds, mutual attachment will result. These mechanisms include visual and postural orientation, smiling, reaching, crying, etc. There seems to be no evidence that food per se operates as a reinforcer of attachment behavior. The principal mechanism involved is a complex interactional choreography of mutual cuing between mother and child. As the baby matures and becomes capable of locomotion, other behavioral systems come into play designed to maintain an optimal balance between proximity and separateness. The infant will cling, pull, grab, and climb on the mothering person, and for every move away from the caretaker there is a corresponding retreat for what Margaret Mahler (1965) has called "refueling." In all of this the baby is quite active, possessing a powerful armamentarium for seduction. The human infant is naturally object-seeking and it experiences acute discomfort until an appropriate object has been found.

Bowlby, who extensively studied the impact of abandonment on infants, has found that the abandoned infant predictably passes through the following behavioral sequence: anxiety, despair, and detachment. Detachment can turn into what Spitz has termed "anaclitic depression," and I am inclined to think of it as the prototype for all human depressions; the baby has lost all hope, it turns its face to the wall, its body temperature drops, and its connection to the world of other humans is all but severed. This sorry state of affairs is not automatically reversed by the caretaker's return; on the contrary, the infant will at first recoil from human touch; it will have to be wooed until it can reestablish the connection. Children differ in their ability to recover from abandonment depressions. Furthermore, the experience itself renders them vulnerable to depressions in later life. If we conceptualize human development, i.e., psychological maturation and growth, as the sequential unfolding of the behavioral systems throughout the life cycle, it then follows that psychopathology must be understood primarily as a form of developmental arrest. In some rare instances that is indeed all it is. Typically, however, the organism makes up for the missing pieces by developing compensatory structures, secondary formations which can range from the merely adequate to the most baroque and sometimes truly catastrophic. Developmentally, we know very little about the origins of manic-depressive disorders, compared to what we know about unipolar depression. Clearly, both mood disorders are multicausal and can originate in traumatic experiences or interpersonal climates at any time in childhood. However, in the etiology of unipolar depression, three major factors, or rather clusters, stand out: (1) abandonment; (2) rejection or abuse; and (3) narcissistic wounds—all of which will be covered in greater detail in Chapter 7.

The fact that depressions, even fatal ones, can occur in very young human infants as well as in animals, clearly indicates that depression can be a more or less total organismic experience. The legacy of Descartes and Hegel still tempts us to think of the human spirit as divorced from the body which contains it. This obviously is a logical fallacy, unless one subscribes to some metaphysical fiction such as an immortal soul which can be divorced from physicality. All that is human about us is contained in our bodies and represents physical events. Unless we understand some of the basic facts and principles of human physiology, the basic behavioral trilogy of mind, mood, and motivation cannot be understood adequately in either mental health or mental illness.

CHAPTER FIVE

The Biology of Cell Communication

Perhaps the simplest and therefore most elegant definition of biology is that it is the science of how cells communicate with each other. How does it happen that the abstract concept of "duty" originating in our mind results in the actual movement of first one leg and then another out of a warm bed and onto a cold floor? What, physiologically, takes place when an acute, painful sensation in a man's chest produces the abstract mental image of the number 911, to call for an ambulance? How can a dream image of a ferocious lion produce a rise in blood pressure and rapid heart beat? In other words, what we would like to explain is how, for example, the concept of work as God-pleasing activity, toil, torture, or whatever, can be translated from an image in the brain—a concept—to a set of actions on the part of the foot, resulting in our getting out of bed on a cold, rainy morning. Conversely, physiological messages from the toe can reach the brain and produce images, thoughts, and feelings of such complexity as, for example, to go searching for a pair of nail clippers to alleviate the pain from an ingrown toenail. Without connections between the brain, mind, and the rest of the body, multicellular organisms could not exist.

What we call mental or emotional processes, thoughts, feelings, affects, and images, are physical events. Otherwise they could not happen. That does not mean that one can be reduced to the other. The mind *is* body; this is not an easy concept to comprehend. This notion of the interwoven nature of the mind-brain entity, as opposed to Cartesian dualism, prompted John Dewey to point out that "only in wonderland can the grin be divorced from the cat." The cat's grin is the subject of this chapter.

If we take the complex task of getting up in the morning, we have an act involving several systems. Assuming that there are no external intrusions other than the fact that the sleeper "knows" that he has to go to work, we can observe a sequence of physiological events that seems to fit the ancient view of the brain and the head as the captain of the ship, giving orders to the crew, which is composed of a multitude of subsystems: cardiovascular, thermoregulatory, respiratory, gastrointestinal, urinary, reproductive, skeletal, and muscular. However, in reality, there is more than just one captain. Instead, there is an ever-evolving triumvirate with democratic tendencies. It can be influenced by its subjects and, in rare instances, it can even be controlled by them.

The brain itself cannot be seen as a rigid and orderly system of different compartments controlling different parts of the body or separate functions. It is an evolutionary patchwork quilt with newer structures superimposed on older ones, comprising three major circuits, and it represents a vast communications network which coordinates the sequence of our actions. What we have is what McLean has termed the "triune brain," which incorporates structures from three evolutionary levels, functionally separable, but acting in concert. The oldest and most primitive is the reptilian brain, which stores and controls the fixed action patterns, what ethologists have called the four f's—feeding, fighting, fleeing, and reproduction. The second set is the mammalian brain, or limbic system, which has been called the seat of emotion. It incorporates, among other functions, the hormonal control system, through the pituitary, thalamus, and hypothalamus. Finally, we have the new mammalian brain (frontal cortex), which in humans is responsible for the most complex mental functions of the brain: thinking and pure reason. Although we can look at some specific feelings or behaviors as originating in one or the other of these circuits, for most mental or behavioral phenomena this is not the case. For example, the smile of the three-month-old baby is the result of a fixed action pattern, and therefore originates in the most primitive, the reptilian brain. Other smiles, however, be they spontaneous or designed to sell a faulty car, obviously involve an entirely different set of brain circuits. The smile of the parents who respond to the baby's smile will do so on three different levels: (1) the greeting in response to another human's smile (fixed action pattern); (2) the joy of parenting (the pleasure centers of the limbic system have been activated); and (3) the happy realization that a developmental milestone has been passed, which represents an intellectual act involving the frontal lobes, which compare an actual event with one described in a book on childcare. Typically, all circuits act in concert with each other and with the rest of the body and they form extremely complex feedback loops.

The neural system controls the organ systems; it represents our communication network and thus coordinates the sequence of actions. We have to get our feet on the floor before standing up, for example, and we have to chew before we swallow. The neural system consists of two principal anatomical parts: the central nervous system, CNS, and the peripheral nervous system, PNS. The CNS is composed of all the neurons within the skull and the spine. It processes incoming information, initiates responses, and sends signals to the organs concerned. The neurons in the brain signal the neurons in the spine, which in turn activate one leg in the direction of the floor. The peripheral nervous system, PNS, comprises all the neurons in the rest of the body. The PNS consists of all the nervous processes that connect the brain and the spinal cord with the sensory receptors, muscles, and glands. Neuroscientists are constantly finding more evidence for the existence of neurons in organs other than the brain or the spinal cord. They seem to be present in every one of the different organ systems, functioning like a multitude of local integrators, a little auxiliary armada.

It should be noted that the neurons in the peripheral nervous system differ from those in the CNS in two important ways: their axons, when cut, can regenerate themselves and, while communication between neurons in the CNS involves more than 40 so far identified or known chemicals, called neurotransmitters, the PNS only uses three. Both the CNS and the PNS act directly on the organs of the body.

The third control system which can also act directly on organ systems is the hypothalamus pituitary complex, the endocrine glands: pituitary, pineal, thyroid, thymus, adrenal, pancreas, and reproductive or sex glands. The hormonal and the neural systems have a remarkable reciprocal relationship, and can excite or inhibit each other. Normally, they act in unison. The central nervous system can signal glands to produce hormones; endocrine hormones, in turn, can stimulate or inhibit specific parts of the CNS. In other words, this interactive system constitutes the neurohormonal control system.

However, the distinction between neural and hormonal is not a neat and simple one, since there exists considerable overlap in form and function. Some neural structures such as the hypothalamus, can *also* function as an endocrine gland, and its action can be neural or chemical, i.e., hormonal. For the most part, the neurohormonal system, the triumvirate (reptilian, mammalian, and frontal cortex) in interaction with the mind, runs the show in concert, forming a multitude of feedback loops of such complexity that the biology student who looks at it for the first time has to conclude that it is a miracle that it works at all, given the millions of possible malfunctions.

In order to understand the nature of the interaction between the neural and the neurohormonal control system and the organism as a whole, we have to shift to the microscopic level of cell communication: the way cells communicate with each other, the means by which they tell each other what to do or not to do, to excite or to inhibit or to reverse an impulse which is both chemical and electrical. The message "get out of bed" literally has to travel from one cell to another, all the way from the brain down to the corresponding cells in the foot: move, do, go. Alternatively, the recognition that a burglar is waiting outside the bedroom door requires the opposite: freeze, play dead, inhibit. The organism has to be able to do all this, with an exceedingly high speed. The runner who suddenly discovers a rattlesnake in his path has to backpeddle very fast indeed. In some instances, such as the one just mentioned, the spinal cord itself engages in a simple decision-making process: fast-freeze, reverse. However, in each instance, each neuron or nerve cell operates in a fashion identical to that of the brain as a whole. It makes decisions in a binary mode. The job of transmitting messages is carried out by the neurons which make up a good part of our brain. They are surrounded by the glial cells whose function it is to carry the waste products of the neurons, to protect them, pass on oxygen and other nutrients, and to act as selective filters. They constitute what is called the blood-brain barrier, and they are of great importance in determining whether or not drugs or other chemicals can reach and influence the brain, i.e., the action of the neurons.

However, glial cells play no direct role in the transmission of neural messages per se. A message starts with a nerve impulse, a momentary change in the conductivity of the cell wall, i.e., in the balance between positively and negatively charged sodium and potassium ions; it then travels inside the cell by electrical transmission. However, to carry the impulse from one nerve cell to another all the way down to its targets, chemicals have to be employed in order to transverse each gap between neurons. Electrical impulses do not jump across synapses. To understand these basic mechanisms, it must be known that all neurons consist of the following components: (1) the cell body (soma); (2) cell membrane; (3) axons; and (4) dendrites (See Figure 1). The cell body, the metabolic center, contains the nucleus and all the necessary machinery for cell functioning. The membrane determines what gets into the cell and what stays out.

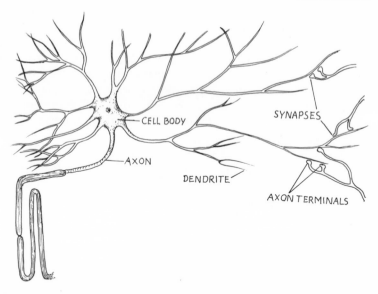

Figure 1. Diagram of a typical nerve cell. Cell bodies for axon terminals (right) are beyond the edge of the diagram.

Since it consists of fatty materials, most water-soluble molecules cannot pass through unless specific gates or channels are opened. Axons are long, thin extensions of the cell body which are designed to carry outgoing messages. They are strictly one-way streets. At their ends they branch out, forming a small bulb-shaped structure called an axon terminal that contains the structures necessary to send the chemical messages across the space between the neurons, which is called the synapse or synaptic cleft (See Figure 2). The axon terminal contains the synaptic vesicles, which store and produce neurotransmitter chemicals, and they contain the mitochondrions which provide the energy needed to release neurotransmitters. Dendrites handle only incoming messages, which means that unless an axon of one cell—A—meets up with the dendrite of another cell—B—(and then C,D,E, etc.) the message cannot be passed on. Meeting up

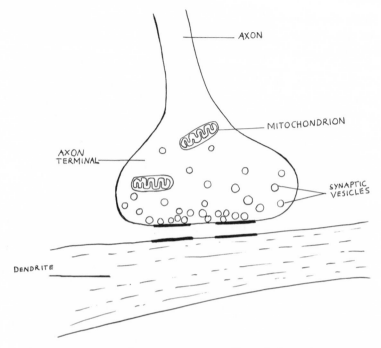

Figure 2. Diagram of a synapse as seen with an electron microscope.

with a dendrite is no guarantee that the message will in fact be passed on. The strength of the impulse has to cross a specific threshold for the cell to fire. The chemicals that are employed for this purpose are called neurotransmitters. The act of writing and formulating this very sentence, including the decision of where to put the comma, probably involved several millions of those electrochemical transactions.

Since the business in the synaptic cleft is of utmost importance in treating mental illness pharmacologically, it is the point of entry, as the processes taking place in the synapse need a closeup. There are already approximately 40 known or suspected neurotransmitters which, obviously, have different chemical compositions and, consequently, different functions.

These substances are stored in the axon button inside synaptic vesicles. When a message from neuron A is supposed to reach neuron B, neurotransmitter substance is scattered across the synaptic cleft, from the proximal end to the distal site, where it attaches itself to the specialized giant molecules called receptors. The receptors in the receiving membrane "bind" the neurotransmitter, which creates a cascade of chemical changes within the membrane, producing electrical potentials. When that event has taken place, neuron B, the postsynaptic nerve cell, goes into action and repeats the process with neuron C. Once the neurotransmitter from neuron A has accomplished its mission, it then has to be removed from the synaptic cleft in order to make room for the next message. This can happen in a number of ways: (1) Reabsorption into the axon or rather the vesicle, a process called *reuptake;* the neurotransmitter can then either be stored or reused, or it can be broken down inside the presynaptic terminal by enzymes; (2) the neurotransmitter can be broken down by various enzymes but inside the synaptic cleft itself.

Different neurons use different neurotransmitters, and to complicate matters even further, some of them have a predominant transmitter and a cotransmitter. Psychotropic drug prescription is an attempt to correct an abnormality in brain functions by intervening inside the synaptic cleft with substances or drugs modulating the production and the metabolism of the chemicals already produced by the brain. In other words, people suffering from mental illness have definite abnormalities in neurotransmitter activity, meaning either too much or too little production, transmission, or absorption. At this point, the neurotransmitters that are thought to be involved in, or implicated as contributing to mental illness, are the following: dopamine, serotonin, noradrenaline, acetylcholine, norepinephrine, and gamma-aminobutyric acid (GABA). The prescribed drugs can do their job in a number of different ways, depending on which part of the system they work on. In this process, which begins with the production (synthesis) of neurotransmitter, and ends with the absorption by the next neuron, a given drug can increase or decrease the amount of the chemical that is produced and released: a drug can attach itself to receptors and thus prevent transmitters from binding (antagonists). It can also mimic it (agonist), or it can change the shape of the receptors making the binding more difficult. Drugs can also work on the enzymes responsible for dissolving the neurotransmitter after it has done its job, thus preventing reuptake and thereby increasing the amount that is available for the next message.

Reuptake agents that are available at present are not entirely specific in accomplishing precisely what they are supposed to do, and nothing else, and furthermore, the body itself, striving to maintain equilibrium, adjusts or reacts to the drug intervention. In other words, psychoactive drugs today are neither the foreign straitjackets they were portrayed, as in popular novels such as Ken Kesey's *One Flew Over the Cuckoo's Nest*, nor are they exact duplications of the substances produced by the human body itself. They are, often at best, approximations, designed to correct chemical imbalances. They can be made into a personalized "fit" with some know-how. Compared to the drugs available as little as 40 years ago, the pharmacological arsenal today constitutes indeed a minor revolution in psychiatry. It is also important to point out, in some instances only, drug treatments today treat the symptoms of depression, not its causes, even though the subjective experience of the patient may sometimes well be that of a miraculous cure. When we speak about "drugs," we are using a term that is exceedingly hazy and imprecise, about as loose a concept as "pet." Is it a cat, a dog, a rat, or a rock? Strictly speaking, a drug is a chemical compound whose mode of action, the how, where, and why it acts the way it does, may be known in its entirety and sometimes not at all. A class of drugs, known as the minor tranquilizers (benzodiazepines, such as Librium) was used successfully for decades before its action was really understood (it took almost a century for aspirin and 30 years for penicillin). Drugs can also have multiple functions and may have different, even opposite effects on different patient populations. The term medication is equally obscure. Caffeine, for example, may be, and very often is, a form of self-medication for a variety of physical and mental ills. So are certain foodstuffs—even food itself. It has to be noted that the most popular nonprescribed psychoactive drugs such as nicotine, and alcohol, appeal to very specific synaptic groups. Hence their use as very dangerous self-medications.

There are a number of ways in which one can classify the drugs that affect the brain and the CNS. The classification system used here, which is meant to be the most general of overviews, is one of *function*, i.e., what they do, what they accomplish behaviorally and experientially.

SEDATIVE HYPNOTIC COMPOUNDS

These act as CNS *depressants*, and include the following: (1) barbiturates; (2) nonbarbiturate hypnotics; (3) antianxiety agents (minor tranquilizers, Librium, Valium, etc.); and (4) others such as alcohol, chloral hydrate, anesthetic gases, etc. All share the following five characteristics: (1) They progressively slow down all the neurons in the CNS, as well as those in the rest of the body. This progression ranges from the relief of anxiety, to sedation, sleep, anesthesia, coma, and finally, death. Death, in this instance, typically results from the arrest of the respiratory system. The effect of these drugs can be either additive: 10 milligrams of Valium is twice as effective as 5 mgs; or the effect can be supra-additive: comparable amounts of one drug, combined with comparable amounts of another drug, can be more than the sum of its parts. In the case of barbiturates and alcohol, two times two may well be 10. A lethal dose of all these drugs alone is usually one that consists of 10 to 20 times the recommended dosage; although, taken alone, i.e., not in combination with alcohol, they do not induce death, even at ultrahigh overdose. (2) There exists an antagonism between depressants and stimulants. As long as a depressant binds a receptor, a stimulant cannot do its work. For example, coffee cannot offset the effects of alcohol until the alcohol has been removed from the synapses. (3) In large dosages, their action is *not* limited to specific neurons, or even regions of the brain; they progressively affect all of them. For example, alcohol works as an antidepressant because, initially, it depresses the inhibitory neurons in the brain and the body—hence the sense of euphoria. In low dosages, all of these drugs reach the inhibitory neurons slightly earlier than the excitory ones. After this initial effect has taken place, depression sets in. Similarly, if a patient with unipolar or bipolar depression is treated with minor tranquilizers, there will be at first a relief from pain, followed by intensification of the depression. The same paradoxical effect occurs when barbiturates are used for the treatment of insomnia. (4) Continued administration of these drugs induces the organism to adjust, which means that sudden withdrawal from the drug does not result in a return to normalcy. Any sudden withdrawal of the drug will result in a "withdrawal syndrome," which includes first hyperexitability, may result in convulsions and, in extreme circumstances, may even result in death. Therefore withdrawal has to be gradual.

(5) If the chronic dosage is high enough it can produce tolerance and dependence, the benchmarks of addiction: the organism needs more of the same substance to accomplish the same results. Furthermore, the liver increases its production of enzymes designed to metabolize these drugs. Some of these drugs can produce cross-tolerance, which means that tolerance for one results in tolerance for the other, and cross-dependence, which means that one drug can be substituted for the other. The minor tranquilizers, a group of compounds known as benzodiazepines, which are anything but minor, were originally designed to replace barbiturates in the treatment of anxiety and insomnia. They were thought to be nonaddictive and relatively harmless, which turned out to be not so simple. In therapeutic dosages, benzodiazepine action is quite specific. It enhances the synaptic inhibition that is mediated by the neurotransmitter gamma-aminobutyric acid (GABA). The minor tranquilizers are extremely effective for the treatment of generalized anxiety dis-

orders, panic attacks, and as a short-term relief from insomnia. They can be used effectively when specific guidelines are applied but should otherwise be avoided. Their side effects may include drowsiness, decrease in short-term memory, clumsiness, impairment of reflexes, and, in some instances, they can release aggression, particularly when mixed with alcohol.

BEHAVIORAL STIMULANTS

These include: (a) amphetamines (Dexedrine, Ritalin, or amphetamine-related compounds); (b) antidepressants (first- and second-generation tricyclics, monoamine oxidase inhibitors, MAOI's, fluoxetine, i.e., the serotonergic agent Prozac), Bupropion (Wellbutrin); (c) cocaine; (d) caffeine; (e) nicotine. In terms of behavioral and mental functioning this group of drugs accomplishes the opposite of that of sedatives and hypnotics: They increase activity, speed up thought processes, sharpen alertness, and they elevate mood. Not surprisingly, they do so in part by mobilizing the neural systems involved in fight, flight, and fright responses. Amphetamines also activate dopamine in two ways: by increasing its release and by blocking reuptake. Since a relative excess of dopamine is a causative factor in schizophrenia, large doses of amphetamines can induce a psychosis resembling schizophrenia in some respects. Amphetamines can exacerbate an existing psychosis or schizophrenic state and they can augment the beneficial action of antidepressants. Caffeine can affect not only the CNS but many organs, such as heart, kidneys, lungs and the arteries supplying blood and *The New York Times* to the brain. Most of these actions seem to be the result of caffeine-induced augmentation of cellular metabolisms. Nicotine exerts its action secondary to a direct stimulation of certain receptors sensitive to the transmitter acetylcholine, which produces increased blood pressure, increased heart rate, release of adrenaline from the adrenal glands, and increased tone and activity of the gastrointestinal tract. For more than a few users it functions as an antidepressant and an anti-anxiety agent. In large doses it can be fatal. Sudden withdrawal can cause in some subjects major mood changes. Amphetamines, cocaine, caffeine, and nicotine are all potentially addictive, which is not the case with antidepressants.

Major affective disorders are thought to result from various imbalances in the relative strength of neurotransmitters, such as serotonin, dopamine, and noradrenaline. Antidepressants, i.e, first- and second-generation tricyclics, monoamine oxidase inhibitors (MAOI's), etc., can address these deficiencies. Antidepressants do not affect nondepressed people although those with sedative properties can make them somewhat sleepy or lethargic; thus they have no recreational value except for those people who are equating sedation with being "high," and they do not usually create addiction or tolerance per se. However, an overdose can be lethal. But if anything, the problem with antidepressants is more typically misuse or underuse, a dosage too low to be effective, which in turn can create a new set of problems, namely the overuse of barbiturates, minor tranquilizers, and alcohol. Proper dosage, i.e., what is called the "therapeutic window," the relatively small range between too little and too much, must be determined with great care. People differ in their metabolic rates and an individual's metabolism can vary with the consumption of other drugs, such as nicotine, which causes these drugs to be metabolized faster.

The side effects of antidepressants tend to vary with their types and the individual's sensitivity. They may include sleepiness, constipation, and dry mouth. MAOI's also require some dietary restrictions.

NARCOTIC ANALGESICS (Opiates)

These include opium, heroin, morphine, and codeine. An opiate is any drug, natural or synthetic, that affects the body in ways similar to those of opium, which is derived from poppy seeds. All of them are extremely effective in relieving pain and diarrhea and in producing euphoria. They are highly addictive because they mimic the effect of substances that naturally occur in the brain. They bind to enkephalin receptors, the receptors for our own opiates, the endorphins. While opiates do not kill the sensation of pain, they change the experience of it into a feeling that exists but one which is not painful. An overdose of opiates can cause death through respiratory failure.

ANTIPSYCHOTIC AGENTS

These include (1) phenothiazines, such as chlorpromazine (Thorazine); (2) thioxanthenes (such as Navane); (3) butyrophenone, such as haloperidol (Haldol). These antipsychotic agents are called the major tranquilizers. They affect the transmission of the neurotransmitter dopamine, particularly in the limbic system. Also, by acting on the brainstem, they suppress certain centers in the behavioral arousal system and thus create in the user a greater indifference to external stimuli. Patients feel less overwhelmed by everything around them. The schizophrenic brain is thought to have too many or abnormal dopamine receptors, a condition which these drugs control but cannot cure. How these abnormalities in the dopamine receptors result in psychotic rambling is not known, nor do we know the obverse, namely how the major tranquilizers control this. When these drugs are administered, the brain initially compensates for their presence by increasing dopamine synthesis. How then do these drugs help? There are several hypotheses to account for their effect: (1) The compensation for receptor blockade is not complete; (2) the increased rate of synthesis and breakdown permits a more precise regulation of the amount of dopamine in each synaptic terminal; and (3) the crucial changes occur in cells that do not use dopamine as a receptor. Since dopamine receptors are concentrated only in certain parts of the brain, neuroleptics, as these drugs are also called, do not "dope up" the entire brain,

but only certain centers. These drugs are nonaddictive and tolerance does not develop. In people who are not psychotic they are
experienced as unpleasant, even as depressants. Their usual
side effects are the so-called extra pyramidal symptoms such as
muscle spasm and restlessness, which can be impressive but
responds readily to anticholinergic drugs. Others include dry
mouth, blurred vision, and a decrease in blood pressure. In
women they can disturb, even block the menstrual cycle and
induce lactation in nonpregnant women. If they are taken in
large doses over a long period of time, the most serious side
effect can be a neurological syndrome known as tardive dyskinesia, consisting of abnormal, involuntary, stereotypical, and
rhythmic motor movements of the face such as puckering, lick-
ing, smacking, and a constant tremor of the lips. The tongue
movement consists of darting, "fly-catcher's tongue," or a pushing out of the cheek, the "bonbon" sign. The occurrence of tardive dyskinesia can be greatly reduced by using low dosage,
switching to different drugs, or by taking an occasional "drug
holiday."

LITHIUM AND ANTICONVULSANT DRUGS

Lithium is used for the treatment of bipolar depression, and
its therapeutic effect can be most dramatic. It works for about
70% of the patients for whom it appears indicated. It is a unique
drug that defies classification because of its multiple applications. It is mostly used in the treatment and the prevention of
bipolar depressions and related conditions such as episodic alcoholism, but it can also prevent the recurrences of unipolar depressions. In addition, it can also be used as a booster for antidepressant medication. Lithium affects both norepinephrine
and serotonin synapses and metabolism, which results in cellular changes that build up slowly over weeks and months. How
Lithium guards against both mania and depression is still a mystery. Since the metabolic rate for Lithium varies a great deal from

one individual to another, even in the same individual over time, blood levels must be monitored carefully to ensure that on the one hand, sufficient amounts are in fact available, while guarding against toxic levels. In excess, Lithium can induce weakness, tremors, fatigue, nausea, abdominal cramps, and diarrhea. Weight gain can occur 30% of the time, as do sleeplessness and lethargy. Most of these side effects disappear after a few weeks, though a slight tremor of the hand may persist. Maintenance therapy requires bi-yearly monitoring of thyroid and kidney functions.

Another class of drugs also has to be mentioned, which has been proven successful as a supplement to or as a replacement for Lithium treatment, namely anticonvulsants. The drugs commonly used are carbamazepine (Tegretol), clonazepam (Klonopine) and Valproic acid (Depakene). Originally, anticonvulsant drugs were developed to treat epilepsy. However, the discovery of their usefulness for bipolar depression was not altogether serendipitous, since the two disorders seem to be related in a certain subgroup of the bipolar population at large.

PSYCHEDELICS AND HALLUCINOGENS

These include: (1) LSD; (2) mescaline; (3) psylocybin (magic mushroom), muscarine (*amanita muscaria* or fly agaric); and (4) substituted amphetamines, D.O.M., S.T.P., etc.; (5) tryptamine derivatives (D.M.T., D.E.T.); (6) psychedelic anesthetics; and (7) cannabis (T.H.C.) (marijuana, hashish, etc.). These drugs, which are reputed to be "mind-expanding" have effects that can range from mild intoxication, to psychosis, to death. Prolonged use can produce both tolerance and cross-tolerance. Dependence is usually more psychological than physiological. Psychosis that has been induced by psychedelics and hallucinogens resembles that of schizophrenia and mania, but amphetamine psychosis is not identical with it in either its clinical picture or its progression.

To measure neurotransmitter activity *in vivo*, particularly in humans, obviously is not easy. However, like any other substances in the body, their metabolites, or their breakdown products, provide an indirect measurement. They appear in the blood, urine, and in the spinal fluid. Furthermore, there are several neurohormonal tests which can reveal abnormalities in the brain-body system controlling both mood and endocrine gland function, and are considered to be putative biological markers for primary depression. Examples are the dexamethasone suppression test (DST) and the thyroid releasing hormone stimulation test (TRH). While at the present time none of them taken alone are conclusive, taken together, and in conjunction with the clinical picture or information, they give a pretty good idea of what course of treatment is most promising. While chemical markers provide one diagnostic approach, measuring the electrical activity of the brain (EEG) and rates of glucose metabolism (PET scan) is another. Quantitative EEG, a computer-assisted measurement of brainwave activity and distribution, using a sophisticated array of statistical analyses, appears to show significant differences between patients suffering from bipolar depression, unipolar depression, schizophrenia, alcoholism, and Alzheimer's disease. Each diagnostic entity seems to have a distinct pattern of brain activity which differs from that of normal controls (See Figure 3).

Considering the rapid expansion of basic and clinical neuroscience, a fair assessment of new technologies is best made by scanning the appropriate literature several times a year. It cannot be captured in a book as basic as this. However, we can still address certain fundamental issues both philosophical and practical, such as how do we know that what we describe psychologically and biologically as a depression in man is indeed what we think it is? The most powerful argument supporting a psychobiological explanation is provided by animal experiments.

When we say that animals and people can die from a broken heart, how do we know that this is not simply an expression of outright anthropomorphism, rather than science? After

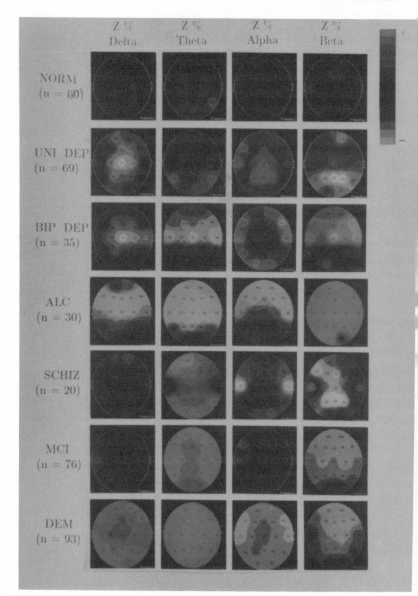

all, a broken heart is a symbolic construct, one which is adjudicated to be uniquely human. Yet, in 1973, Jane Goodall reported on a sequence of events from her studies of chimpanzees in Tanzania. One of the females of the group, called Flo, died. One of her sons, Flint, showed all the signs of grief and depression. He looked and acted dejected, he stopped eating and relating to others, and finally he was found dead in the exact place where he had last seen his mother. An autopsy revealed that this young healthy male had succumbed to a viral infection which normally is quite benign. While it makes sense to *interpret* this event as Flint having "died of grief," this is still only suggestive evidence, not in any way empirical *proof*. To substantiate that the psychological and physiological mechanisms involved are similar, if not identical, we need experiments which show that the psychosocial stresses assumed to cause depression in humans will have the same effect on animals *and* that the therapeutic measures required for the treatment of humans also help animals. In other words, the models employed in such experiments should resemble the conditions modeled in etiology, biochemistry, symptomatology, and treatment. Experimentally, that represents a tall order. Yet, the evidence accumulated so far, is quite impressive:

1. Learned helplessness: Animals exposed to uncontrollable stress will exhibit performance deficits in subsequent learning tasks which are absent in animals who have experienced identical stresses but were able to control it; for example, exposure to electric shock that the experimental group could not control, while the control group could. The experimental group learned that nothing they did would be effective; consequently, they passively endured all subsequent shocks. They were unable to learn, later, that by jumping a bar they could control that same

---

←

Figure 3. Examples of a quantative EEG. From John, E.R., Pricep, L.S., Fridman, J., & Easton, P. Neurometrics: Computer-assisted differential diagnosis of brian dysfunctions. *Science*, 1988, *239*, 162–169. Copyright © 1988 by the American Association for the Advancement of Science. Reprinted by permission.

shock. The helplessness effect has a considerable degree of generality; it applies to cold water immersion, underwater immersion, as well as to purely cognitive tasks such as visual discrimination and experiments with uncontrollable noise. The effect of these experiences in animals can be reversed by the application of antidepressant drugs. The animals in the experimental groups showed all the signs of psychomotor retardation, a prime symptom of endogenomorphic depression. In some other experiments it was shown that the helplessness effect could also be mediated by forcibly exposing the animals to the fact that responding, i.e., jumping the bar, does result in termination of the electric shocks. Inescapable shock leads to depletion of catecholamines in the brain, while controllable shock does not.

2. Behavioral despair: Closely related to learned helplessness, it requires animals to swim in confined space. After a period of frenzied attempts to escape, they will assume a posture of immobility. In subsequent immersions the onset of immobility happens more rapidly. However, pretreatment with a wide range of antidepressant drugs will delay this response, i.e., the onset of immobility.

3. Chronic unpredictable stress: In this case, animals were exposed to a variety of different stresses, such as electric shocks, water immersion, reversal of light and dark cycle, noise, and bright lights, all of which significantly lowered the animal's subsequent ability to deal with new stresses. However, the animals who received antidepressant drug treatment during the period of chronic stress showed no such impairment. There is by now quite a bit of evidence that in humans, chronic low-grade stress is at least as potent, probably even more so, in precipitating depression than the acute stress generated by traumatic life events.

4. Separation: Infant monkeys respond to maternal separation first by protest, i.e., agitation, sleeplessness, distress vocalization, followed by despair, i.e., decrease in activity, appetite, and social interaction. These behavior patterns closely resemble the state of anaclitic depression in human infants that has been

observed by Spitz and Bowlby. Furthermore, the separated monkeys showed significant changes in their pituitary-adrenal activity, which in turn responds to antidepressant treatment.

5. Incentive disengagement: Rats trained in a runway for food rewards were switched to nonreward training. After an initial increase in agitation and corresponding increase in activity, behavioral depression set in. Willner (1985) has hypothesized that these incentive experiments explain the mechanisms by which depressive reaction to separation operates in humans, namely by lack of social reinforcement and social support.

6. Intracranial self-stimulation: In this group of experiments, electrodes were implanted into the reward system of the brains of animals, thereby raising the threshold for reward responses. Withdrawal produced depression which in turn responded to antidepressant medications which returned the threshold to its normal level. These findings provide evidence for those theories of depression which implicate reductions in the activity of the reward systems of the brain as a principal cause for depression.

On the whole, modern psychoactive drugs do a quite adequate job in controlling the symptoms of the major mental illnesses. Sometimes even a short-term application will permanently reverse a depressive episode, and sometimes the patient merely becomes functional as opposed to being a candidate for the backward of a mental institution. The person functions at less than 100% of his potential, struggles with assorted side effects but, given the alternative, this is still a major improvement. There are manic depressive illness reports of patients who climbed out of the hell of with the help of Lithium, took it for the rest of their lives, and never encountered another problem. I have no scientific grounds on which to dispute such claims. It is only that my own patients have not yet been this cooperative. I have, however, encountered an occasional patient (see the case of Mary in Chapter two) who sadly experienced the opposite: After an initially good response to drugs, the patient began to deteriorate for no apparent reason, teetering on the edge of a breakdown until, again for no discernible reason, she improved. We hypothesize in this case that when Mary was first medicated, she was experiencing the beginnings of a major, fairly autonomous neurohormonal change, one which is taking its course. Pharmacologically it could be slowed down, but it could not be reversed. However, such cases are the exception rather than the rule. It has to be noted that the majority of patients with mood disorders can respond to appropriate dosages of medication with improvements that range from merely better to more or less symptom-free. Given the range of possible medications and possible side effects, the newness of the specialty of psychopharmacology, and the speed with which new discoveries in diagnosis and treatment are being made, my own professional preference for choosing a physician to medicate my patients is always one for whom this particular aspect of the therapeutic work is his or her *major* line of work and of research interest.

However, in the case of dual treatment, the question can be raised: what effects do the fact that there are *two* people working with the same patient have on the nature of the transference? Obviously, every patient reacts differently. Some responses, though usually of short duration, are quite common: (1) The physician, adjudicated to be the magician, is idealized, while the therapist is devalued. If they also happen to be male and female, respectively, the magician does the real work, while the female therapist merely changes the diapers—just like home; (2) The physician is devalued as the "drug pusher" while the "real" analytic work is done in therapy. If that is the case, the patient may feel that it is of vital importance that medications be discontinued as soon as possible; (3) Both therapists are devalued, one as being helpless to fix the problem verbally, and the other as just one more fad. Generally, however, once these stages, singly or together have been resolved, the arrangement has worked very well. What is more, the power of the transference, the power inherent in the therapeutic interaction, with its entirely unequal exchange of information, combined with the power of the subscription pad, taken together, to this therapist's mind, represent more power than any one human being should be entrusted with or burdened by.

I also believe that, before we can discuss the concept of psychobiology, it is important to examine some methodological issues. During the last decade, readers of such publications as the science section of *The New York Times*, or of *Psychology Today*, published by the American Psychological Association, not to mention the media in general, have been bombarded with headlines such as "Nutrition Linked to Emotional States," or "Vitamins Associated with Depression"—in other words, headlines linking a multitude of substances or physical states with moods or mood disorders. These studies typically involve "correlations" or "relationships" or "associations," which to the unwary reader suggest cause-and-effect relationships, when, in reality, they prove no such thing. Correlations can be tricky indeed: for example, a detailed, longitudinal study of the coastal towns of Schleswig-Holstein in northern Germany found statistically highly significant correlations between the number of storks in any given year and the number of babies born. Unless one accepts the obvious explanation—the one "everybody knows," namely, that storks bring babies—one has to look for the variable that connects these two findings or data by either predating both (antecedent variable) or by causally connecting the two variables or sets (intervening variable). In this particular instance the antecedent variable was "good and plentiful crops," which, in rural societies traditionally correlates with increases in birth rates. Crops are also associated with the population of frogs, which are a staple of stork life. While it is quite clear how the greater availability of foodstuffs increases the number of organisms who have to live off it, it is a much more complicated interaction that explains the correlation between crops and birth rates. In the first place, more frogs feed more storks who survive to make more storks, who in turn. . . etc. In the second instance, we have to explain how the abundance of food makes people beget more babies. Do good crops simply make farmers more optimistic, grateful to God, sexy, or does this Thanksgiving syndrome mean that availability of food affects such diverse factors as sexual activity, fertility, generalized health, and decrease of the proportion of stillbirths and infant mortality? A fictitious headline such as "Scientists Discover Relationship between Barley Production and Human Lactation" or "Wheat Production Deepens Christian Faith," would miss the point in more ways than one, because it arbitrarily, though accurately, connects diverse points of a complex psychobiological and sociobiological network. Keeping in mind that every correlation and/or cause-and-effect relationship in this area should always include in parentheses the notation "typically" or "on the average," we can sort out a number of probable cause-and-effect relationships, which are subject to a vast number of modifiers—for example, food and fertility. Starvation inhibits ovulation, and semi-starvation affects the entire reproductive cycle in terms of the probability of success.

Semi-starvation also causes depression along a strictly biological pathway. If semi-starvation is the product of oppression or that of continued failed effort—despite all attempts the crops failed again, despite backbreaking labor, religious fervor, countless sacrifices and prayers, etc., the draught persisted—the resulting semi-starvation may cause demoralization which lowers sexual desire and probably the chances for impregnation. The same number of calories consumed by a society with high hopes and visions for the future will probably not have an appreciably lower birthrate. A rural family struggling with survival is highly motivated to produce as many children as possible, since every surviving child is a potential farmhand. But if infant or maternal mortality, due to the scarcity of food resources, exceeds a certain point, fertility rates drop sharply. There is just so much grief humans can deal with and still maintain their desire to procreate. Furthermore, the finding that substance A is related to feeling state B also tells us very little about the relative weight of substance A compared to other factors. At first sight this statement seems obvious. More or less of any substance in organisms of comparable size and comparable states of health or unhealth ought to have a greater or lesser effect. But that is not necessarily the case for a number of reasons, some of which we understand, others of which we do not. For example, some heavy smokers feel little or no negative effects on their moods when they quit, while others suffer terribly and may even succumb to a depression. Nobody knows yet exactly why this should be so. Strangely enough, the most persuasive explanations for this phenomenon have been provided by philosophers (e.g., Jean-Paul Sartre and Hans Martin Gauger). What we do know are two things: One, the mind which "frames" the biological experience can quite powerfully determine how the body reacts, and two, there are innumerable fail-safe mechanisms built into the system that are designed to correct imbalances. In fact, they are so exquisite that one could argue that the real question is not why a given imbalance is correlated with a specific unwelcome or painful emotional state, but what it is about the organism so affected that prevented the regulatory system, physical or mental, from springing into action in the first place. On very rare occasions, seemingly small irritants to the system can wreak major havoc. While sharks rarely sink battleships, jet planes, which have no trouble flying over the North Pole, can be brought down by a bunch of birds who get sucked into their propellers. Such incongruous outcomes are rare; they usually involve a complex chain reaction where the failure of one system ushers in the failure of the next, etc., until the entire organism breaks down temporarily or permanently. This can happen to the neurohormonal control system. The acute onset of mania is an example. It constitutes a biochemical emergency that has to be addressed first. Otherwise the organism might self-destruct. In terms of relative weight, a fullblown attack of mania probably resembles that of a hurricane which makes the stress-resistance of the hull of any ship caught in it an entirely academic question. Any ship will sink if a tidal wave is powerful enough.

In mood disorders, as in almost all other human affairs,

causality typically means a complex interaction of probably more factors than we can ever hope to know.

Looking at homo sapiens as a primarily symbolic animal, and having an increasing understanding of functional neuroanatomy, obviously raises the question: How do they relate to each other? That is the point at which psychobiology and sociobiology, together with a few other life sciences, enter the picture. We are the product of evolution, but we make our own world. Obviously, no definitive answers are attempted here, merely the joy of demonstrating that for every psychological research finding there is at least one biological one, and vice versa, which do not contradict each other but, more often than not, generate a stream of mutual paradigm adjustments.

CHAPTER SIX

Psychobiology

The Interaction between Our Symbolic World and Our Evolutionary Inheritance

In genetic and evolutionary terms homo sapien is an omnivorous higher primate with the capacity for social learning and for abstract thought. Our genetic makeup, the basic model, is that of the hunter-gatherer who began to populate this globe about 10,000 years ago, a time span far too short for natural selection to have accomplished any significant genetic changes. These 10,000 years represent merely a tiny percentage of evolutionary history. Consequently, our fundamental biological blueprint, determining cognition, thought, and behavior is still the same as it was then and as it still is in all societies, be they Western or the so-called primitive tribes which still inhabit the more remote regions on this planet. In that sense, the Australian aborigine is no different from homo Americanus. This blueprint constitutes what Melvin Konner (1982) has called "the biological constraints on the human spirit"; it defines the limits of our ability to adapt and, at the same time, to ensure the survival of the species. To use the simplest of examples, we can, up to a point, adapt to certain climates—the tropics, subtropics, and what we call the temperate zones. In the regions beyond that we have to rely on our ingenuity in building fires, constructing habitats, and producing and wearing protective clothing. Otherwise we would die from the cold.

When we say that a given trait or behavior is genetically determined, what exactly does that mean? First of all, we assume that the gene responsible for it exists because at some point in time—or maybe even for the most part—it was useful and advantageous for reproductive success—the basic principles of evolution, one so basic that it prompted some genetic biologists jokingly to define a person as "just a gene's way of making another gene." First of all, the fact that a trait was once useful does not mean that it still is, nor that it is necessarily advantageous. It also does not indicate whether the trait or behavior is good or bad, nor how compatible it may still be with the conditions of today's postindustrial society. Some of our genetic inheritance is an outright nuisance. Depression is a prime example; so is schizophrenia. The same is true for our patterns of food consumption. Our metabolism is geared towards the diet and the lifestyle of our cave-dwelling ancestors which means two things: one, the composition of their meals, its food value, relied primarily on carbohydrates, grains high in fiber and low in animal proteins and fats; and, two, since scarcity of food has been the rule in almost all of human history, our organism is geared towards the storage of energy in the form of fat, in order to survive the inevitable lean times. Thus, biologically, we are predisposed to what in a food economy of plenty constitutes unhealthy overeating. Staying slim in this day and age does not come naturally at all. We have to choose between loving carrots, exercising regularly, or living with a low degree of hunger most of the time.

Secondly, the fact that something is "genetic" does not mean that it will necessarily happen. Sometimes it does, and sometimes it does not. For example, a child who has one or both parents with brown eyes inherits at least one dominant gene for that color and therefore the child will be twice as likely to be born with brown eyes than with blue ones. Then there are instances where even a minor change in a molecule of DNA, a single gene mutation can produce changes in chemical reactions in a behavioral control system of the organism, resulting in dramatic behavioral or cognitive changes, which override all the predetermined cognitive systems. For instance, PKU (phenylketonuria), a severe form of mental retardation, is the result of such a single-gene mutation. But it will only occur if the fetus has inherited a double dose of that abnormal recessive gene. At the same time, a simple change of diet, after birth, the elimination of a single, specific amino acid, can successfully counteract the deleterious effect and expression of that gene. These instances, however, are the exception. Generally, we have to distinguish between the degrees of heritability, which means two things: one, the probability of inheriting a given trait; and, two, the degree to which the gene will in fact dictate a given trait or behavior. For example, Huntington's chorea, a neurological disorder with onset in midlife, which causes intellectual deterioration, psychosis, and abnormalities of muscular functioning, is entirely genetically determined. In this instance, gene equals behavior. In the case of human intelligence, on the other hand, genetic endowment and environmental stimulation are both of importance, perhaps even in almost equal measure.

In the case of fruit flies we essentially know the whole line of development from gene to behavior. In humans we know it completely in some instances, vaguely in others, and not at all in most. Typically, what we inherit are predispositions, whose actual manifestations are contingent on a vast number of concurrent factors. We now know that in the schizophrenias and in the case of affective and panic disorders, genes are very important. For example, in identical twins, the concordance rate for depression, i.e., the probability that if one of them has it, the other one will get it too, even if they were raised apart, is estimated to be 50%. For fraternal twins and ordinary siblings the rate is also the same: 10%. For bipolar disorders the estimates range from 50% to 80%. The rates for schizophrenia, for first-degree relatives is 10–20%, as opposed to 1% in the general population.

While those odds predict risk, it is also important to note that the risk factor is never 100%. We have yet to explain the cases where genes predispose an individual for mental illness, but where it fails to develop. The fact that the lifetime risk for major depression is 20–26% for women, 8–12% for men, and at least 2–5% for bipolar disorders for both sexes, raises some very intriguing questions. Why is it so common? Why does it exist at all? What evolutionary advantage, if any, could it possibly have had? Obviously, traits that carry a disadvantage are rapidly bred out, unless the trait only manifests itself after the animal has had a chance to procreate. Heart disease is an example of a condition that typically develops after the organism has reproduced. It can therefore be passed on to the offspring. Shortsighted pigeons, on the other hand, would not be likely to find enough food and therefore would probably not survive long enough to reproduce. In addition, the manifestation of a trait may be very different, depending on whether one or two of a particular gene are present. For instance: one sickle-cell gene provides a degree of immunity to malaria, while two of the same gene results in sickle-cell anemia, a debilitating and usually fatal disease among American blacks. Immunity to malaria in Africa was highly advantageous; in America it was not necessary, in the absence of the malaria-carrying mosquito.

While I do not mean to imply that all—nor perhaps even most—genetically determined traits exist because they necessarily were advantageous, an interesting theoretical question nevertheless is what such advantage might have been. After all, evolution is governed by both order and chaos. Psychobiology and sociobiology should not be confused with a particular *branch* of sociobiology which, by substituting evolution for God, and fiction for fact, ended up with some fairly baroque claims about the inherent "wisdom" in all biological phenomena.

With respect to the evolutionary advantage of genes for mental illness, the following theories have been proposed:

Schizophrenia may be a manifestation of a genetic phenomenon called "polymorphic balance," i.e., the variability of the gene pool which ensures a greater range of adaptability to changing environments. While this may or may not be true, it still does not answer the question why the incidence of schizophrenia is as high as it is, and why that has been so constant throughout recorded history, regardless of the culture in which it occurred. With respect to mania and depression we are on much firmer ground. The dependent young must have mechanisms that increase the chances of survival in case they are separated from their mother and the group. Distress vocalization, initially, increases the chances of being found and rescued. However, it soon becomes dangerous for several reasons: it attracts predators and it uses up energy that is needed to survive without food and warmth. Playing possum is an extremely valuable action pattern for energy preservation and for escaping unwanted attention. If all somatic and vegetative functions slow down, if the body temperature drops, the animal pup or the human baby can survive for a much longer time. Generally, there are times in life when it pays to lie low, for example when recovering from a major loss, or when the environment consistently frustrates one's effort. A period of reduced effort and energy output allows for recuperation and a rethinking of possible directions. Conversely, mania can be to one's advantage if resources are scarce and when a great deal of energy is required to acquire necessary foodstuffs. If one has a limited amount of time to prepare for a disaster, such as a hurricane, a little mania can be exceedingly useful. Moreover, it has been suggested (Price, 1967; Gardner, 1982) that in animal hordes and in human groups having a strong hierarchical order, individuals, passing through the different stages in the hierarchy, have to be able very suddenly to increase or decrease their energy output. The transition from follower to leader requires a sudden surge, and the displaced leader of the pack has to suddenly submit, subordinate himself, stop fighting, and throw in the towel.

As inherited action potentials, the capacity for both feeling states are advantageous, since in our evolution we passed through a stage in which small social groups were regulated by a strict dominance hierarchy, similar to those in baboons and macaques. For their stability, hierarchies require certain behavior patterns from their members, such as irritability towards inferiors, anxiety towards superiors, elation on going up in the hierarchy and depression on coming down. Because of the great survival advantage which they provided for the group as a whole, these behavior patterns may well have been selected. Clearly communicated social ranks in animal groupings have the following advantages: they reduce the frequency of intragroup fighting, aid the defense of the group against others, enhance cooperative efforts in food-gathering, and protect reproductive patterns. What that means is that even though there is no obvious animal analog for manic-depressive disorder, there probably exist for all social animals distinctive neurophysiological "organismic" states that underlie behavior patterns correlated with social position. For example, McLean (1971), watching rainbow lizards fighting for leadership, observed: "Twice we saw dominant lizards defeated and humiliated . . . they lost their majestic colors, turned muddy brown, became depressed and died two weeks later" (Hooper Teresi, 1986, p. 46). People with bipolar disorder, according to Gardner (1983), exhibit an overly sensitive onset trigger and a pronounced *insensitivity* to those reactions that would normally stop an animal from continuing to display a given posture. The lack of feedback from the presumed followers does not turn off the behavior. In bipolar patients that very lack of response may worsen the condition because to be imbued with the conviction of being the appointed leader of the pack, without response from those potentially led, produces a dilemma. Where are my adoring masses, and why don't they applaud? It is this dilemma to which an individual reacts with a stress reaction, denial, projection, paranoia, and other primitive or psychotic defense mechanisms. While this is a fascinating hypothesis, strangely, there has been no follow-up research either to confirm or to invalidate it.

The next question then, it seems, is: How important are genes in determining human traits? Humans differ from animals only in the degree to which their behavior is genetically determined, "wired in," as computer language would have it. Prior to birth, genes determine where cells go and what functions they shall have. The neurons in the brains of animals at birth are predominantly committed to a set of functions, such as distinguishing between bugs and nonbugs, for instance; there are hardly any cells available to incorporate experience. In humans there are also portions that are wired in, but they constitute a much smaller percentage of the overall number available. If we look at the different spheres of human behavior, certain observations have been made. For example, if we examine some of the most basic spheres of human behavior and interaction, we observe the following:

1. *Procreation.* Genetically we are programmed to mate, and most of us, to procreate. How, when, where, and with whom is left to choice. Animals too show wide ranges of mating patterns, but for each species that particular pattern is a biological given and subject to fairly limited variation. The same is not true for humans: in 83% of the 849 societies studied by George Peter Murdock in 1967, one man was married to two or more women (polygamy); half of those do this on a regular basis and the other half do it occasionally. Only 16% of societies examined by Murdock practice monogamy—one man married to one woman. Marriages between one woman and several men occur in only 0.5%, and in contemporary Western society serial monogamy—one or several exclusive marriages or other forms of living together and raising offspring, seems to be becoming the rule. Additionally, the homosexual population is estimated (or rather, guesstimated) to range from 5–12% in most societies. Mating and procreation, then, are not necessarily connected. For human procreation to succeed, all that is needed is for an egg and a sperm to unite, and for environmental conditions to enable the embryo to survive. The various cells, as they multiply, know what to do, regardless of whether they are in a human womb or not and regardless of whether or not the womb in

question is biologically related to the fetus, or even whether or not it is human.

2. *Sex*. What constitutes sex and gender is determined by chromosomes, hormones, and experience. All human embryos start out as biological females. However, the release of specific amounts of particular sex hormones in the uterus at very precise times during the embryo's life determines whether the infant is born a male or a female. A genetic female develops into a biological female automatically; she requires no additional hormonal prompting. Genetic males, in contrast, require exposure to male sex hormones, particularly testosterone, in order to become biological males. A genetically male fetus, deprived of testosterone, the male sex hormone, will biologically develop along female lines. The baby will be born as a genetic male, but one with the reproductive organs of a female, with only the most rudimentary and undeveloped male organs. Variations in hormonal exposure in utero and at different critical points in fetal development can produce varying degrees of androgyny, some of which are reversible, while others are not. Androgyny (degrees of hermaphrodism) among humans involves sex and sex-dimorphic behavior, including cognition and temperament. There are instances where due to faulty hormonal mechanisms a genetically female fetus can be exposed to male sex hormones. For example, a single-gene recessive defect can result in the fact that the enzyme steroid 21 (hydroxylase) production is insufficient. As a result, not enough of it is available to do the job of transforming progesterone into cortisol. Because of this deficiency the pathway of cortisol production is blocked. Instead, the hormone enters a different production path, taking place in the gonads, which leads to the production of testosterone and other androgens, masculinizing the fetus. Even if that defect is corrected at birth, the girls who were born with it were, at age 10, more tomboyish, engaged in less doll-play, and less inclined to say that they wanted to marry when they grew up than their normal controls.

3. *Gender*. Sex alone determines neither gender identity nor

gender roles. Experience as a modulatory factor does that for the most part. In the nuclear family, whether or not a biological male will experience himself as a male or as a female depends on whether or not, psychologically, the male can move beyond the primary identification with the female caretaker, a process that Robert Stoller (1968) has called "disidentification," the mechanism through which the boy relinquishes that primary identification, which then allows him to identify with and to incorporate male role models. If the mother, through subtle but nevertheless powerful enough signals, prevents this process from taking place, the boy will not be able to actualize the existing maleness level (as determined by the testosterone impregnation index in utero). If that takes place the boy is likely to become a transsexual, i.e., someone who "knows" himself to be a female with the same degree of certainty with which normal biological females know themselves to be unquestionably of the female gender. This is called "core gender identity." Thus, originally, at least, gender seems to be truly in the eyes of the beholder, the primary caretaker.

How universally true are we to regard these findings by Stoller and colleagues? For example, Imperato-McGinley and coworkers (1972) reported 18 cases of male pseudohermaphrodites also due to an enzyme deficiency in utero, where the babies were born with a scrotum which appeared labia-like, and with a very small phallus, who appeared to be primarily female and who were therefore raised as girls. At puberty, however, that hormonal imbalance corrected itself, the children developed into normal males with male sex organs, a deepening of the voice, phallic growth, and a generally male body build. Of these 18 youngsters, who in the Dominican Republic where they were found are commonly referred to as "penis at 12," 16 changed their gender identity to male, one remained female, and another switched to a male identity but continued to wear feminine clothing. While at first these findings seem to cast doubt on Stoller's claims about the relative importance of sex assignment and upbringing versus the influence of postnatal androgens, that changes considerably if the following variables are examined: The fact that these children in terms of sex and gender were recognized as belonging to a distinct and different entity (penis at 12), the recognition on their part and on the part of their caretakers and peers that physiologically they were not normal females suggests that they were not raised unambiguously as females. What these findings do indicate, however, is that human beings, under specific and unusual circumstances, are capable of changing their gender identity relatively late in life.

4. *Sex dimorphism.* In more general terms, applicable to all animals, sex dimorphism, the famous difference between the sexes, is determined by several variables which are related to mating patterns and the ecological context within which they take place. The latter may call for what in evolutionary biology is known as an R-strategy (rapid and prolific breeding), or a K-strategy (restrained and slow, nearing the carrying capacity for a given habitat). Secondly, in species where one sex invests more heavily in the rearing of the young, in terms of ovulation, gestation and infant care, the investing sex becomes a limited resource for which the other sex competes. In those instances sex dimorphism with respect to body size, body build, and aggressive potential, is pronounced. Males aim to copulate indiscriminately, while females do the opposite, mating selectively, reserving as much energy as possible for the raising of the young. To the extent, however, that males are involved in the rearing of the young, pair-bonding is required. In those instances we find low levels of sex dimorphism in terms of body size, levels of aggression, and territoriality. Males in that case are not free to choose their strategies but must mold them to the needs of the female for the rearing of the offspring. Dominance and status are important for both sexes, for the males to be successful breeders and for the females to be successful mothers. For the female, status determines access to energy resources. Consequently, high-status females begin their reproductive lives earlier, bear more offspring, have their births

more closely spaced, have more infants that survive, and bear earlier in the birthing season.

The energy cost of lactation for the mammalian female has been estimated roughly to equal that of the male needed for the defense of the territory, competition for females, and for providing food (Ehrhardt, 1985). Human sexual dimorphism in terms of body size, stature, and muscularity, i.e., the anatomy of the aggressive potential, is relatively minor by mammalian standards. One of the major differences between males and females lies in the ability to store energy in fat deposits. That ability, in turn, determines the sequencing of pubertal events and the establishment of fertility. For menstruation and ovulation to take place, more than 10% of body weight has to be fat, in other words, enough to provide the energy for one year of lactation, which is one of the reasons anorectic girls regularly suffer from amenorrhea. This has had important ramifications for the evolution of human intelligence. Human milk is uniquely suited for the growth of brain tissue as opposed to muscle and bone, since it is extremely low in proteins and high in lactose and lipids. This is so important because during the first year of life 65% of the metabolic rate of infants is devoted to brain growth and only 8% to that of muscle. In contrast to rhesus monkeys whose brains at birth have already grown to 68% of their adult size, the human brain at birth constitutes only 23% of its adult size. However, it completes 93–95% of its growth in volume by the end of the fourth year—the usual age of weaning among hunter-gatherers. In other words, there are powerful biological-evolutionary forces at work to ensure that the postnatal brain is properly nourished during the period when the young organism is at its most formative in terms of developing those qualities that render us specifically human.

Behaviorally, then, as Alice Rossi (1985) has put it, "gender differentiation is not simply a function of socialization, capitalist production or patriarchy. It is grounded in a sex dimorphism that serves the fundamental purpose of reproducing the species" (p. 161). The major psychological differences between males and females that are rooted in biology occur in the following spheres: (1) sensory sensitivity; (2) aggression and general level of activity; (3) cognitive skills (spacial, quantitative, and verbal skills); and (4) parenting behavior.

5. *Hormones and behavior.* The female, focused on child rearing, is naturally more affiliative, has a greater commitment to and involvement with the community and the environment. Men, in contrast, are less affiliative during their younger years, ages 15 to 25, when their testosterone production and corresponding levels of aggressive energy are at peak. During the reproductive years in men, the influence of hormones on behavior is at its highest. Testosterone production correlates with social deviance such as crime, sexual violence, alcoholism, drug abuse, etc. Our society, particularly among the poor where there is an increasing trend towards female parenting without a male partner, thus excludes males from the restraining influence of babies. It is now a generally accepted proposition that the human infant is born with an imperative need for attachments; it thereby automatically issues an invitation to bond. Those interpersonal cues could counteract, at least to some extent, the aggressive and competitive component of the human male, if social life offered him a chance to be exposed to it. Add to this lonely psychobiological configuration the psychological and biological correlates of growing up male, such as having to find one's niche in society, vocational opportunities, or rather the absence thereof, changes in self-concept, physical strength, and inclination towards risk-taking behavior, then, all taken together, they result in a gender gap of such magnitude that it prompted Gaston Bouthol (1969) to propose that the size of the pool of unattached, unemployed, substance-abusing, angry men in their late teens or early 20s, constitutes one of the best predictors of impending war. Whether this is in fact accurate is open to question. That this particular population constitutes a powerful and potentially dangerous force to be reckoned with is not. After all, his group of humans typically provides the populations that make up the largest part of most armies and they

constitute the majority among most prison inmates. On the whole, among people and animals, pair-bonding and intra-species violence are inversely correlated. What that means is the following: The more the males are attached to their females and actively involved in the raising of young, the less likely they are to fight with each other. Conversely, to the degree that they copulate competitively, do not exist in pairs, the more likely they are to attempt to kill each other and whoever else gets in their way. To quote Melvin Konner: "Men in groups or in packs are not very nice." The question of whether sexual dimorphism among humans is good or bad is really moot; biologically it is central for both production as well as reproduction. While the central importance of sex dimorphism for reproduction is obvious, the same cannot be said for its importance for production, which traditionally has been associated with male characteristics. However, when Spence and Helmreich (1978) correlated male and female characteristics with scientific productivity as measured by objective standards, it turned out that those scientists *high on both the masculinity and the femininity scales* were the ones most scientifically productive. Biological sexual dimorphism is part of the genetic package that we share with the hunter-gatherers; it is a given: its relative weight in determining the behavior of individuals and groups and human affairs in general is an entirely different matter. I will return to it later in this chapter. First we need to reexamine the three basic behavioral systems: attachments, sexuality and parenting.

In all primates attachment behavior is an inborn behavioral system. All neonates are therefore naturally "object-seeking," i.e., in search of an object to attach themselves to. This impulse is so powerful that it overrides almost all other behavioral systems. It is not dictated by need satisfaction, such as for love and food. As Harlow (1971) has shown, infant monkeys develop attachments; given a choice between a wire surrogate model that provides food and a cloth surrogate that does not, the monkeys consistently chose the cloth model to cling to. Moreover, when clinging behavior to the cloth model was punished by blasts of cold air, it increased rather than decreased the monkey's clinging. Negative reinforcement does not work in this instance. In fact it achieves the opposite result. Konrad Lorenz (1958) has shown a similar mechanism operating among ducklings.

Given the choice between an animal of a different species or no live nurturing object at all, humans and monkeys will gladly accept cats, dogs, and other mammals as substitutes, and they will fare fairly well with them. Babies who fail to thrive can be partially rehabilitated by pets who choose to adopt them. Intraspecies interaction of so profound a nature is not restricted to the relationships between the very young. While it is, for example, known and not at all uncommon that women who were unable to conceive have become pregnant shortly after they adopted a child, there have also been cases of women in the same predicament who took a puppy, and raised it with all the care given a baby, which seems to have produced the hormonal changes necessary for conception. Puppies can in fact make babies.

As mentioned earlier, the flip side of attachment behavior is separation anxiety which, if not alleviated, will traverse the behavioral sequence of protest, despair, and detachment. Another important behavioral system entails the impulse to explore the environment and the impulse to play, which includes sexual play. Juvenile sexual play—including sexual mounting—is universal among monkeys and apes; it is part of what Winnicott (1965) has called the "normal expectable environment," without which the genetically encoded innate responses and fixed action patterns, even those most crucial to reproduction, would not emerge normally. Harlow's (1971) motherless rhesus monkeys were unable to figure out how to copulate: they literally did not know where or into which part of the female anatomy to put their penis. During this crucial period of social learning, play is not an idle pursuit; it is a vital exercise in trying out adult roles, acquiring interactive patterns, and for the development of cognitive functions. Sexual play, which is part of the exploratory behavioral set, is originally directed at the mother who diverts it towards siblings and peers. Among hunter-gatherers the sexual drive propels the youngsters towards autonomy—away from the family. The transition from hunting and gathering towards farming and agriculture, when children had to be kept for the family to survive as an economic unit, produced a push-pull situation: towards and away from the family and, correspondingly, Oedipal attachments. In that sense, as Bacciagaluppi (1982) has argued, the Oedipus complex is really a pathological, secondary structure, the result of a double bind—be autonomous, but don't go away.

Parenting, the third vital behavioral system, is also inborn—waiting for the baby to function as a releaser. However, the degree to which it will materialize in action is contingent on the proper unfolding and the development of the earlier organizers of the psyche. In that sense, parenting behavior is both totally genetic and entirely environmental. Parenting is instinctual, but it must be learned through the experience of having a parent or substitute parent, and by practicing on peers—quite a delicate balance.

Another important area of inquiry pertains to the relationship between hormones and behavior. Behavioral endocrinology has provided us with impressive and powerful empirical examples of hormonal influences on behavior. Prenatal sex hormones and their influence on gender are a prime example and, as such, indisputable. However, we have not yet addressed in general the question of the relative weight of biological variables in human affairs. Hormones influence behavior; but that does not necessarily mean that they determine it: The way in which the mind experiences—frames—the physiological manifestations of a hormonal event, may well determine what the individual ends up actually feeling and experiencing. This line of investigation began with a by now well-known experiment by Schachter and Singer (1962) in which the investigators tested the role of perception on the subject's experience of the effect of epinephrine, one of the stress hormones. This chemical substance causes physiological arousal, i.e., heart palpitation, muscle tremor, and skin flush. One group of subjects was informed correctly of what the effects would be, while a second one was told the exact opposite. They were led to believe that they would experience numbness in their feet, itching, and headache. The third group knew nothing about the possible effects. Finally, to make sure that the epinephrine, in the dosage administered, had any effect at all, a fourth group was given a saline solution. One-half of each group was then subjected to either an annoying and angry-making treatment by a confederate of the researcher or, alternatively, by a playful and euphoric one. The placebo and the informed groups were relatively unaffected by the emotional climate created by the assistants. However, the uninformed group experienced the emotions the researchers had been trying to induce. The findings concerning the uninformed group as compared with those of the placebo group and the informed group indicates that arousal, i.e., the stimulating effect of the epinephrine, is a prerequisite for a heightened emotion, which explains why the placebo group did not have much of a response. However, the uninformed subjects felt *something* that needed an explanatory frame: "I am feeling this way because . . . the researcher makes me feel happy/angry. . . . my physics exam was harder/easier than expected," etc. Any reasonable cause that can label and explain the sensation of physiological turmoil becomes acceptable as the cause, as the "truth," for the subject who experiences it. By differentiating arousal from emotion, it shows that at least this particular hormone need not be specific in its emotional effect. Depending on the context in which it is produced or administered, it is still the human mind that has to do the interpreting of its meaning as being good, bad, or indifferent. While some scientists still regard these findings as somewhat controversial, they nevertheless opened the door to a very exciting line of research. An equally intriguing line of inquiry deals with the impact of social interaction on hormone production, and vice versa. For example, the relationship between testosterone and serotonin on the one hand, and dominance and competition on the other. Testosterone increases aggressive behavior in males, and it naturally rises and falls with the degree and amount of aggression that the organism expresses. Velvet monkeys, who were made to fight with each other, first showed an increase in testosterone levels and a corresponding decrease when they stopped fighting. However, in later comparing the testosterone levels of the winners with those of the losers in these fights, the losers showed a significantly lower level of testosterone than the winners. Research with members of the Harvard wrestling team showed variations identical to those of the velvet monkeys. Levels of serotonin, a neurotransmitter, also correlate with dominance in velvet monkeys. Dominant monkeys have the highest levels, soldiers have the lowest. When the dominant male is removed from the colony his serotonin level drops, while the animal who replaces him shows a corresponding increase *until* the chief is returned to the group and to his accustomed position. Dominant males assert their position twice per day through dominance-display signals. When the boss flexes his muscles, looking appropriately stern, all his subordinates jump to attention. However, when the chief was made to exercise his display of dominance behind a one-way mirror where he could see his troops, but they could not see him, his posturing, obviously, could not have any effect on them. The experience of being ignored by his subjects, of feeling totally impotent, resulted in an immediate and significant drop in serotonin levels in those dominant males deprived of a following. It seems that in velvet monkeys and among college students, serotonin levels correlate with machismo.

The serotonin connection becomes even more intriguing when we look at its relationship with violence and suicide. Serotonin levels (as measured by the metabolite of serotonin 5-HIAA in the spinal fluid) correlates with random violence. The levels of serotonin among homeless hoodlums was comparable with the low serotonin levels found in low-status monkeys, which indicates that random aggression is the obverse of dominance, which makes sense, since fear and rage physiologically exist on a continuum (fight and flight) and both involve the activation of the body's general stress response. The boss does not have to fight—he only needs to signal to get the desired response. Fairly timeless forms of teenage violence, only recently renamed as a phenomenon called "wilding," have always been an expression of powerlessness, disenfranchisement, and alienation. Dominant monkeys whose serotonin levels were artificially lowered became hostile, nasty, bitchy, and slightly crazy. Not surprisingly, 5-HIAA can be an extremely accurate predictor for suicide. M. T. Asberg (1976), at the Carolinska Hospital in Sweden, found a high correlation not only with suicide but also with the means to accomplish it. The lower the 5-HIAA level, the more violent and therefore effective the means of suicide. Statistically, an average of 2% of the people who have attempted suicide, but have survived, will succeed in killing themselves within the course of one year from the attempt. However, given low serotonin levels, the proportion of suicide survivors who will end up dead in the same space of time jumps to 20%. However, it is also important to note that low serotonin levels have also been found in people who have never been depressed, or, for that matter, violent. Obviously, serotonin then is only one of many mood-regulating factors, but one which apparently is important enough for specific populations. Furthermore, the only study of a suicide epidemic in a mental hospital, where suicide rates had previously been extremely low (see Chapter Three), showed that the decisive variable was *hope* or, rather, the degree to which the significant persons in the environment communicated *their own* loss of hope with respect to their ability to help those particular patients. What was even more surprising is the fact that when the investigators explored the instruments employed by those suicidal patients in their initial attempts, the investigators found that some of them were derived from suggestions made by the staff. For example, the depressed patient who was put on suicide watch and was asked to surrender his eyeglasses protested vehemently. In response, he was given the explanation that the lenses could potentially lend themselves to the purpose of cutting his wrists. The patient, who had never thought about his glasses as having any other function but to alleviate his myopia, ended up doing precisely that. What Lionel Tiger (1979) has termed "the biology of hope," from the little we know about it empirically, seems to center around the presence of opiate peptides—endorphins—produced by the brain. Taken together, the research on the role of hope and that on brain chemistry poses an important challenge for further psychobiological research. For example, if we examine the phenomenon of self-mutilation, i.e., the fairly common occurrence of people who repeatedly feel compelled to cut, burn, or otherwise disfigure themselves, we have several seemingly contradictory explanations for this strange behavior. As a religious ritual, it has been practiced for at least as long as man has left records of his activities. With respect to its intrapsychic functions it can represent a simple affirmation of existence: I cut, I bleed, I hurt, therefore I am real, visible, I exist. In that way it may be a defense against psychotic disintegration. Alternatively it can be an expression of self-punishment. Interpersonally, particularly if the injury is dramatic and in a prominent place, it lends itself to the purpose of the sadistic manipulation of other people, be it to get attention, to indict, or to punish the other person. However, the fact that self-mutilators experience the act as soothing, and that they rarely feel any pain, could prompt the question whether this act is not simply designed to activate the production of endorphins in order to counteract an acute depression. This view is supported by the fact that this expression of pathology is particularly common among bipolar patients, where it may well represent an attempt to actively initiate the switch from depression into mania. On the other hand, one could argue, if the sensation of acute, intense pain and a corresponding rise in endorphins was the only purpose of that exercise, it could be just as easily inflicted on body parts that are hidden instead of obvious. What is more, pain that causes no visible injuries at all could be inflicted, such as putting one's finger into a light socket. In other words, the impact of the wound on a real or imagined onlooker must clearly be of importance. What is more, of all social institutions, prisons have the highest incidence of self-mutilation, a fact which plays havoc with the bipolar-endorphin hypothesis. If, on the other hand, we subsume all of these explanations under the category of control—intrapsychic, interpersonal, or in terms of mood and its biochemistry, the contradictions pretty much disappear. By damaging themselves, self-mutilators exert a small measure of control over circumstances that are experienced as overwhelming and all-controlling.

Further along the line of inquiry into mind influencing biological events, even overriding seeming biological imperatives, a few more examples are the studies which examined women, living under dormitory conditions, who wound up inadvertently, unconsciously coordinating their menstrual cycles. It seems reasonable to hypothesize that the same may be true for testosterone levels among men in groups, which could further explain the ferocity of victorious armies and the fact that among young men, gang rape is much more common than one-on-one rape. Voodoo death has been documented in many different tribes. The conviction that a taboo has been violated, that a powerful spell has been cast, will indeed result in death, one that is ascribed to rapid shifts or fluctuations between activity of the sympathetic and parasympathetic nervous systems. People can will themselves to die.

Hypnosis is another fascinating example. With some patients it has been used in surgery as a substitute for local, even general, anesthesia. In fact, some of the leading experts on the subject, such as Ernest L. Rossi (1985, 1986) go so far as to claim that hypnosis—an apparently mind-related phenomenon—can move not only molecules in general but also molecules on the genetic level. Under stress, the limbic-hypothalamic system converts neural messages of the psyche and the mind into the neurohormonal messenger molecules of the body. This we already know. But Rossi goes on to say:

> These (messenger molecules) in turn, can direct the endocrine system to produce steroid hormones that can reach into the nucleus of different cells of the body to modulate the expression of genes. These genes then direct the cells to produce the various molecules that will regulate the metabolism, growth, activity level, sexuality, and the immune response in sickness and in health. There really is a mind-gene connection! The mind ultimately does modulate the creation and expression of the molecules of life! (p. xiv)

While this powerful claim has yet to be put to rigorous empirical testing and validation, the potential analgesic power of hypnosis alone demands that this avenue be explored very seriously indeed. At this point we have some hypotheses with respect to what the mechanisms are that are responsible for the pain-suppressing actions of acupuncture, electrical brain stimulation, and the placebo effect, namely the activation of endorphin production. The placebo effect has been estimated to work for about 50% of all psychoactive drugs if given acutely. Rossi (1986) claims that includes tricyclics and Lithium, a claim that has yet to be demonstrated to occur *over time*. The fact remains—the belief that a given drug will have a specific effect can make it a self-fulfilling prophecy. The mechanism which is responsible is the activation of the natural opium production of the brain, the group of neuropeptides called endorphins. Candace Pert (1986), in a series of fascinating experiments with radioactive naloxone, an opium antagonist, unequivocally demonstrated that the placebo effect, which by definition is "all in the mind," can be turned on and off by endorphin-blocking drugs such as naloxone. Receptors, blocked by naloxone, cannot bind brain morphines.

Now, if we return to the problem of sex dimorphism once more, the biologically given difference between males and females, we know that they exist universally and we know that they play a role and that they influence behavior and cognition, up to a point. But what is their *relative* importance compared to the impact of socialization? Alice Rossi argued convincingly, and subsequent research seems to confirm this, that some kind of "compensatory" education or learning in early childhood can and will mitigate the undesirable aspects of sex dimorphism. In other words, socialization geared towards remedying the cognitive and interpersonal shortcomings of both sexes in childhood can make up for biological predisposition. For example, while animal research has shown that it is possible to invoke nurturant behavior towards the young through the administration of female sex hormones to virgin prepubescent males and females, it has also been shown that males not given those hormones will show nurturant behavior if they are simply exposed to pups for a long enough period of time. Hormones may prime an organism for the display of nurturant behavior, but it still takes continuous proximity for the display to be exhibited and maintained.

Finally, the research on survival under extreme situations is another area where the reciprocity of thoughts and physiology are striking. On the one hand, longitudinal studies of concentration camp survivors suggest that the experience resulted in significantly higher rates of incidence for physical and mental illness, a psychobiological configuration that can be loosely subsumed under the term "posttraumatic stress disorders." On the other hand, if we examine the literature on what determines survival in the first place, it seems quite clear that in this situation which, psychologically and physiologically, must have been one of the most stressful experiences any human can endure anywhere, then all things being equal, the variable with the greatest predictive power in forecasting survival was not a physical-biological one, but the absence or presence of a belief system. People who were able to maintain the hope that their suffering made sense, that eventually it would benefit somebody, that God had a reason to allow this to happen, that it might hasten the advent of communism and/or democracy, that rescue was imminent or at least inevitable—in other words, any mental construct that sustained the will to live—could mobilize the organism to somehow adapt to the torturous assaults on mind and body. Inmates turned into what was called *Muselmaenner*, people who adopted a demeanor and appearance that indicated that they would die shortly, when their belief system could no longer sustain them, when they had lost hope. In fact, Thompson (1981) has stated unequivocally that given identical physiological and psychological stresses on the body and the neurohormonal control system, nonhuman organisms—animals—are *more vulnerable* than humans. The research evidence seems to indicate that this difference is *not* due to the fact that biologically we are sturdier organisms—we are not—but to the fact that humans can acquire an arsenal of coping mechanisms to counteract stress. We can dream, we can concentrate on a vision of the beach while enduring the dentist. Lionel Tiger (1979) has argued persuasively that hope is as much a part of human nature as our need for sex and food, that it is as necessary for survival as air, given the uncertainties of life and the certainty of death. It is quite likely that the evolution of the human cortex favored the development of a talent for imagination and optimism to counteract the demoralizing effects of defeat, death, famine, and sickness. Optimists are more likely to cope with adversity in an unpredictable environment and, therefore, are more likely to reproduce than pessimists. Besides the development of a cortex which can envision a future with chemicals such as endorphins which facilitate the redistribution of energy is necessary to maintain effort and belief by anesthetizing the organism against the pain and failure, and supplying the energy for renewed efforts. These opiates "stimulate a social and psychological state which augments the animal's survival chances under circumstances in which a cold and correct assessment might be sufficiently demoralizing to mean the difference between life and death" (Tiger, 1979, p. 169). Put differently, the fact that humans are capable of devising and exercising mental "tricks," such as wishful thinking, illusions, together with our infinite capacity to fool ourselves, while causing us a lot of grief and making up a good part of the workload of psychotherapy, is also extremely adaptive, since it represents a very necessary tool for survival.

The Acquisition of Mood Regulation in the Human Infant

In order to understand what renders the human organism vulnerable to depression, we have to examine how mood and mood regulation normally develop in infancy and early childhood. Most of the existing theories about the etiology of depression have been derived from the analysis of adult patients who, together with their analysts, reconstructed the events that may have contributed to the development of a particular mood disorder. Stern (1987) refers to that entity as the "clinical infant," as distinguished from the "observed infant," a construct which has been arrived at from the actual observation of normal and not-so-normal children. In what follows we will discuss primarily the observed infant and those inferences about its affective and cognitive structures that have been developed from these systematic observations and that are congruent with the data of ethology. The section of this chapter which deals with case history material naturally has to discuss the clinical infant.

The human baby enters life with a blueprint for its psychological and physiological development, together with an entire arsenal of behavior patterns, or systems, designed to elicit mothering behavior from a primary caretaker, and a powerful need for secure attachments. Michael Balint (1968) has termed the basic orientation of the infant towards the world "primary love." The mother-child dyad, together, negotiates an interaction designed to allow for the gradual unfolding of the baby's potential, the realization of its intrinsically social nature. According to Thompson (1981) the baby is born with a set of affective behavioral groupings, recognizable by muscular responses: surprise, startle, interest-excitement, enjoyment-joy, distress-anguish, anger-rage, fear-terror, contempt-disgust, and shame-humiliation. Each affect is conceived of as being controlled by an inherited program of neuronal firing which, in turn, controls not only facial muscles, but also autonomic blood flow, and respiratory and vocal responses.

During the first three to four years the infant has to traverse the entire route from birth with only a "sense of core self" (Stern 1987) to an autonomous little person who exists separate from, even in opposition to, other humans and objects. Margaret Mahler has called this process "the psychological birth of the human infant" (1965). During this time span a multitude of developmental tasks has to be accomplished, most of which require interaction with another human or humans. The human environment acts as the facilitator—one which should be optimally attuned to the inner world of the infant and the signals through which it communicates. The emphasis here is on the *mutuality* of the interaction. For example, if we compare the situation of the human infant with that of the black bear cubs, in terms of early mother-child interaction, it is dramatically different. In the case of the bears, the litter is born while the mother is hibernating. The process of giving birth barely rouses her from sleep. The cubs are born blind; they migrate to the nipples by sensing heat, an entirely autonomous movement on the part of the offspring. For the next three months they stay enfolded in a warm pocket made by the mother's curled-up sleeping body. During that period the bonding process takes place without any active input on the part of the mother other than the passive supply of milk and body heat. The human infant, in contrast, from the beginning, is exquisitely attuned to and dependent on every nuance of the affective and cognitive interaction with its caretaker. For example, the baby will react to perturbations in emotional attunement between mother and child as early as the age of two months. The mother who suddenly becomes still-faced or impassive in the middle of a social interaction with the child, will produce a mild upset or withdrawal on the baby's part. The infant "knows" that in the exchange it has been left hanging, so to speak, and it will react. Conversely, the infant can also say a decisive "no" to the caretaker; it can assert its independence by gaze aversion.

In terms of biological heritage, the contemporary baby, which is still the hunter-gatherer infant, is geared towards on-command feeding as often as every half-hour, and it is also primed for continuous physical proximity. Infants were typically carried in a sling by their mother during the day and they slept with their mothers at night. During the first three months physiological regulation is the major adaptive task to be negotiated (Sander, 1964). Distress signals have to be understood and responded to. The mother must learn to distinguish between a hunger cry and one which is due to other causes, such as pain, cold, loneliness, separation anxiety, etc., a common misunderstanding between a colicky baby and its mother. The distress originating in the intestinal tract is mistaken for hunger, i.e., distress coming from the stomach, and responded to with feeding which in turn causes more gastric disturbances, thus establishing a vicious cycle of despair and helplessness in both members of the dyad. In a similar vein, the baby will respond to maternal overstimulation by turning its head to the side. An insecure mother may interpret this as a rejection and respond with hurt or rage; a potentially tragic misunderstanding.

At birth the infant has very few means of self-soothing, and only few means of self-stimulation. The organism, immature as it is, requires very specific conditions in order to mature. Besides food, it needs rocking, being walked, cooing, changes in light and dark, noise and quiet, and temperature regulation. All these interactions are necessary not just for psychological well-being but for physiological maturation as well. Important neural pathways, an archaic form of memory and learning, are laid down, sleep patterns are established, and the infant's metabolism in general adjusts to extrauterine life. In that respect, the immature organism is entirely dependent on a caretaker for stimulation, protection from overstimulation, and for soothing. The communication during the first months of life between mother and child consists of signs from the infant and signals from the mother. The kinds of signals that the baby "understands" are: equilibrium, tension (muscular or emotional), posture, temperature, vibrations, skin and body contact, rhythm, tempo, duration, pitch, tone, resonance, and probably a number of others which the adult is barely aware of. Eventually, the human infant learns the means of self-soothing and to entertain itself, but only if it has had a chance to enjoy and to internalize these mothering functions from a caretaker. In the area of mood regulation it is important to distinguish between the inborn "sets," which are mostly defensive in nature, and the input from the environment. The infant can defend itself against overstimulation, which can be due to either abandonment or maternal intrusiveness, by simply "shutting down," but it has as yet no means available which would allow it to take active steps in the direction of making itself feel *better*. The baby is born with organizing mechanisms that can store, sort, and retain "good me" and "good object" experiences, which then can slowly turn into a repertoire of self-soothing behaviors and symbols. Heinz Kohut (1971, 1977) has called these processes "transmuting internalizations." The sounds and feelings of being comforted are something the infant takes into itself through repeated experience and eventually these memories are something the child can call forth in mother's absence. The intermediate step is the acquisition of transitional objects, things such as a security blanket, a doll, or a pet which are imbued with the magical qualities of the caretaker. The transitional-object stage is the halfway step between absolute and concrete dependence on the one hand and symbolic and abstract representations of the internalized parent, on the other.

Frances Lear (1989), an accomplished editor and a bipolar depressive, recently recounted in a way that was most moving, how her first step out of a severe depressive episode was the recall or the memory of herself as a person who once before recovered from depression. From the memory that a recovery *had* taken place she moved on to the actual process of *how* she actually accomplished it. She then essentially followed her own footsteps out of her previous episode, starting with changing the color of her dress to one her mother had particularly liked on her. "Piece by piece, I gathered up my whole self, as if it was a string of pearls, and returned myself to me. . . . On that long-ago evening, I understood at last that the tiny voyage I had just taken—which seemed to me a thousand treks to the moon— would someday be less arduous, would perhaps be like riding the gentle dips along the ocean's shore. Yes, I was certain of it. There was medication to stabilize, and the past to let go" (p. 144).

One of the key concepts of self-psychology is that of the "self-object" (Kohut, 1977), which means that one organism utilizes some or all parts of another organism as functional parts of the self: either "me as part of mother," or "mother as part of me." "Together, as a unit, we are capable of negotiating the world." Another way of looking at that same (hypothetical) process is to see it as a functional symbiosis between two brains, since the infant's brain and central nervous system are far from self-sufficient (Basch 1975). There is a very good reason, for example, why at birth the mother automatically puts the infant at her left side, where her heart is, because she thereby attempts to restore to the infant the familiar prenatal connection with her cardiac rhythm. In a similar vein, mother's brain remains the auxiliary agent for the ordering function of the infant's cerebral cortex for optimal stimulation and as a filter for noxious stimuli and as an aid to information processing. The concept "self-object" has to be distinguished from that of "self-object representations." The latter are interactive, interpersonal, cognitive, and affective units, comprised of memories of how we experienced mother's affective response to us, that become internalized and as such have a powerful influence on the formation of the self. The infant which is left too much to its own devices, or abandoned, loses much more than simple company or security. It loses necessary interactive ingredients for physiological well-being and for mood regulation. Such infants will literally "fail to thrive," become depressed, develop marasmus (a gradual loss of flesh and bone characteristic of malnutrition) and a variety of other deficiency syndromes. What is more, abandonments in early childhood predispose children to depression in adult life every time these adults have to deal with abandonment, rejection, or death. The initial reaction to abandonment is protest (in response to separation anxiety), followed by despair (which is related to grief and mourning), followed by detachment (which is the dynamic of an anaclitic depression). This primitive defense will be readily encoded into the immature brain as part of its behavioral repertoire for dealing with future abandonments.

In order to reach "psychological birth" the child has to change from a body that registers hunger merely as organismic distress to a being separate and mature enough to say, "I am hungry," and "I want food;" in other words, it has to develop a sense of self. Developmentally, Stern (1987) distinguishes between (1) a sense of core self, the experience of a physical self which is coherent, willful, and unique; and (2) a subjectively experienced sense of an "emergent self" (from birth to 21 months). This represents the shift from existing primarily in the eyes of another to primarily being for the self. Between the second and the sixth months the interaction with "other selves," i.e., entities not coexistent with the self, alerts the child to the fact that mother and child are quite separate physically, that they are different agents, have distinct affective experiences, and separate histories. With these realizations the infant enters what Stern calls the "domain of core relatedness." Later, between the age of seven and nine months, the child discovers another new subjective perspective, namely that there are other minds out there. This new sense of a subjective self conveys the possibility for a much more complex interactive field, namely intersubjectivity between caretaker and child. The interaction between two subjectivities, two realities, ushers in the "domain of intersubjective relatedness," a quantum leap from core relatedness. Now, mental states can be read, matched, aligned with, attuned to or, alternatively, mismatched, misread, misaligned, or misattuned.

Eventually, the signaling ability of the infant becomes the precursor of language, the emergence of a verbal self, the "domain of verbal intersubjective relatedness." Only then can the child begin to be able to grasp the concept that "a sweater is a garment a child has to put on when mother starts freezing." In other words, the child learns that mother and infant do not necessarily experience reality in the same way and that at times mother's reality will be superimposed on its own. With the advent of upright locomotion everything changes dramatically because glory and shame enter the picture forcefully. For the first time the infant entertains the brand new notion that it, the child itself, can be the initiator of separation: it can walk away and it can return. This phase, which Margaret Mahler has called "Separation and Individuation," consists of four subphases: (1) Differentiation (six to 10 months): the child discovers locomotion and it zestfully approaches the environment for pleasure and stimulation. The toddler has "a love affair with the world" (Mahler). Mother ceases to be the sole center of the child's universe. (2) The practicing period (10–18 months), upright locomotion, exploration, and the development of representational intelligence all contribute to the child's inflated grandiosity. Nothing in later life, including the winning of the Nobel prize, ever makes us feel as good about ourselves. Visually, the whole world changes, simply because the vertical, the upright look at objects changes all the angles. Besides, distant objects can be brought close by approaching them. (3) Rapprochement (16–24 months): all grandiosity notwithstanding, the toddler learns that he is still a dependent and relatively helpless little person. The child's attempts to balance independence and separation anxiety result in a gradual deflation of his grandiose sense of self. In this crucial phase the toddler vacillates between needing to explore and wanting to stand on his own two feet and the imperative for refueling, i.e., a sudden return to mother for additional emotional supplies. During this particular time, a mother has to strike quite a delicate balance between overprotectiveness and unavailability in order to prevent either premature disillusionment or premature separation. (4) The fourth subphase (roughly the third year), is characterized by the unfolding of the more complex cognitive functions and verbal communication patterns, etc. By the end of the third year, psychological birth should be complete—if all went well—the toddler has become a little person in its own right. During the practicing subphase, the infant discovers itself for the first time as the agent of highest elation (if not mania) and of glory, by standing up; as well as the agent of the most profound deflation, depression, and shame, by falling flat on his face or rear end. The possible pitfalls for the child during that part of the development are the potential consequences of parental mirroring, applause, mockery, or shaming, in terms of its ability for mood regulation, the capacity to deal with failure and deflation in later life. For example, one of the most powerful little cartoon strips that just about every German child grows up with depicts the ridiculous spectacle of a frog climbing a tree. He is clearly imitating a bird and so far he has succeeded. But, this morality tale informs the impressionable reader that if the frog assumes that he also knows how to fly, he will learn a painful and humiliating object lesson in presumptuousness. Having landed flat on his belly, the mockery of the superior adult rings out, *"Who do you think you are?"*

Since the concept of intersubjectivity is so central, not only to the understanding of early childhood development, but also to that of psychopathology and psychotherapy, we have to look at it in greater detail. Contrary to what Freud thought, the human infant is not born with a built-in stimulus barrier. Unless it is protected, internal perturbations and external stimuli, stresses and impingements threaten the psychobiological well-being of the baby. A "good enough holding environment" as Winnicott (1965) has called it, is one that reads the baby's signals correctly most of the time. The baby "learns" that crying brings relief sooner or later. The mother, as a person, as well as an "environment," constitutes for the baby what Masud Khan (1974) has called "the protective shield." Without it the baby would be overwhelmed by all the stresses it encounters and it would be unable to mature. What Spitz has called "the organizers of the psyche," are principles of organization which help the child to make some sense out of its chaotic environment. These organizers of the psyche are the mechanisms through which affects are linked to cognition. The three-months' smile, the social smile, is an expression of happy recognition, and therefore a reward for the caretaker. The stranger-anxiety at eight months, however, indicates that the child now perceives a *mismatch* between expectation—the familiar face of the parent—and reality—the alien face of the stranger. An experience of mismatch is both unpleasant and frightening. The organizers of the psyche must then be understood as affectively loaded mental file cabinets. They are needed by the infant because random events have to become ordered experiences, raw feelings must be shaped into proper emotions, brute sensations have to be organized into clear perceptions, and random impulses must become guiding purposes. For this to take place the baby requires a human mirror, someone who confirms, plays back, validates, repeats, orders and, most importantly, helps to alleviate those sensations that are painful.

For example, for the simple equation—pain equals bad—to become a meaningful association would be quite difficult if the caretaker's response to the infant's expression of pain alternated between utter delight and deep concern, or if the baby's signals of distress evoked anger on the part of the mother sometimes and resulted in soothing behavior at others. If responses would be this inconsistent, the baby would be reduced to a permanent state of behavioral despair. Its symbolic world would be severely impaired. The sense of self, both with and in opposition to other selves, the interface of subjective and objective self, would be entirely chaotic. Basic behavioral symbolic sequences, such as pain leads to crying, which results in being picked up, which feels soothing, or a hunger-cry leads to feeding, which results in satiation and then sleep cannot become secure elements in the experiential world of the infant. Similarly, simple equations such as "me equals good, equals a gleam in mother's eyes," experiences which constitute the basic building blocks for self-esteem, have to be exercised over and over again until they become a solid part of the self. This level of core relatedness or that of "basic fault," as Balint has called it, the stage of "primary love," is where the baby needs a good enough symbiosis with a primary caretaker. What the baby wants is to "be able to love in peace" (Balint). Normal maturational processes propel the infant from a secure, symbiotic attachment towards separation and individuation and, eventually, in the direction of genuine autonomy. Disturbances during this crucial stage, psychotoxic elements in the interaction such as this list compiled by Spitz (1965) will result in lasting vulnerabilities and worsen preexisting genetic vulnerabilities: (1) overt primal rejection; (2) primary anxious overpermissiveness; (3) hostility in the guise of anxiety; (4) oscillation between pampering and hostility; (5) cyclical mood swings; (6) hostility consciously compensated for with reassurance and, finally; (7) partial or complete emotional deprivation. A "fault line" originating during the first year of life is likely to cause later psychopathology given specific amounts of similar stresses. The extent to which it in fact develops depends on, among other things, whether or not there were enough other beneficial factors, i.e., alternate caretakers in childhood to compensate for it. The terms "good enough mother," "affect attunement," "interaffectivity," and "empathic responsiveness" all refer to the same thing: namely, one (usually mature) organism understanding another (immature) organism and the former being able to respond appropriately to the latter.

Obviously, not all mother-infant dyads manage this equally well. Several things can go wrong. Besides outright misattunement, i.e., the total inability on the part of the mother to understand the baby's signs, a mother can be selectively attuned, understanding and responding to some but not all of the child's messages. A mother who is ill at ease with her own sexual and animalistic impulses and who has disavowed them in herself, will have great difficulty with such messages from her baby. Conversely, a caretaker may be overattuned, exhibiting a form of psychic hovering over the child, that can be experienced as quite intrusive. The mother who is overidentified with her infant and unconsciously aims to repair damage that was inflicted on her, the mother, during her own childhood, is likely to absorb each and every psychic utterance from her child. Such intense scrutiny on the part of a parent can profoundly interfere with autonomy and privacy. The mirror image of the type of attunement offered the child on the part of the primary caretaker becomes the prototype for the kind of attachment which the child will develop with subsequent partners. Attachment per se was long thought of as a developmental task of a particular phase in childhood (Bowlby, 1958, 1960). That line of inquiry, however, neglects the quality or the "style" of attachment or bonding. Research has shown that the type of attachment developed in the original caretaker-child dyad, unless corrected, tends to extend through life. It is replicated in our relationships with friends, peers, spouses, and, later on, with our own children. Ainsworth *et al.* (1978) distinguishes between three basic types of attachments: (1) secure; (2) anxious/avoidant; and (3) anxious/resistant. It appears that the quality of the relationship at the age of one is an excellent predictor for the quality of relating up to the age of six. Anxious attachment patterns at the age of 12 months are predictive of psychopathology at age six. Predictively, the patterns persist into adulthood among middle-class Americans. Though it seems plausible that this should be true for other cultures as well, cross-cultural studies have not succeeded yet in substantiating the universality of these inter-relationships.

Before turning to the particular depressogenic factors and, specifically, to the influence that a manic, depressed, or bipolar parent can have on a child, we have to first examine the transition from early attachment to autonomy, the concept of an ambivalent symbiosis, and that of a malignant symbiosis and, correspondingly, that of a developmental arrest (Searles, 1965; Bacciagaluppi, 1982). It has been suggested by both authors that a bad, malignant, or ambivalent symbiosis may well be at the core of all psychopathology. A satisfactory or good enough symbiosis ushers in the phase of individuation and separation and then psychological birth. What happens in the case of an ambivalent or malignant symbiosis is a two-phase frustration. During the symbiotic phase the mother does not meet the child's attachment needs, or she outright rejects them because of her own frustrated dependency needs which render her unattuned to the needs of her infant. Once the child reaches the developmental stage of individuation, however, she keeps the child bound in a pathological symbiosis. While during the earlier stage, her own repressed dependency needs prevented her from giving to the child—she wants to be the one who is given to—likewise, she is unable to let go of the child when that becomes age-appropriate. Now the deprived baby in herself wants to be given to by her own child. She then feels threatened by abandonment when the child achieves autonomy. On another level, she may envy its autonomy because she had had to sacrifice her autonomy to the needs of the toddler. Tragically, the human infant is programmed to cling to the caretaker, regardless, even if the caretaker herself is the source of the infant's frustration or pain. In the wilds, this type of ill-treatment of the young was a more remote possibility. Consequently, evolution did not evolve any genetic-biological safeguards against this event. In an ambivalent symbiosis there is never a resolution, since the child can never be what the mother wants it to be, namely a mothering figure. Mother never gets what she wants either, and therefore, she never can let go. The child, in this instance, enters into a bargain; it sacrifices its own dependency needs in the hope of getting them met eventually. Since this too never happens, the child also stays bound to its mother, forever disappointed and perpetually hoping for a good, or at least better symbiosis.

If we equate psychological maturation and psychological health with the unfolding of the behavioral, cognitive, and affective blueprint with which we are born, a less than optimal or good enough environment will selectively prevent this process from taking place. Maturational events that should take place do not happen. In that respect, all psychopathology may be at first merely a developmental arrest. A good example for such an archaic or retarded formation is what Kernberg (1978) has described as the defensive mode of "splitting." In terms of cognitive development the small infant is incapable of dealing with either ambivalence or ambiguity. What that means is that, as far as the child can tell, an object is either all good or all bad. In that sense we can conceptualize (hypothetically), that the infant may have the subjective experience of having two mothers and two selves, one good and rewarding, the other frustrating and painful. To attribute both good and bad aspects to the same object requires a degree of cognitive maturation for all infants that does not develop until the end of the second year. A child who experiences excessive frustrations will not mature appropriately, and therefore it may not develop the capacity for the tolerance for ambivalence. Such children, as adults, present an almost identical clinical picture in the way in which they respond to interpersonal frustrations. From one moment to the next the friend, who up to that point could do no wrong, suddenly becomes an untrustworthy, terrible person, bearing no relationship to the earlier, idealized version.

However, while the concept of a developmental arrest is extremely helpful and necessary, it is also usually not sufficient. The parts of the person which were prevented from developing often require the formation of compensatory structures in order to make up for the missing parts and in order to accommodate pathological parental demands or conditions. The most extreme form of defense against mistreatment and inappropriate demands is perhaps the formation of a multiple personality. Alternatively, the child who is prevented from developing a sense of basic mastery over the environment would be doomed to despair unless it can find some other way to accomplish things. It could be argued that one way of understanding the psychopath is to see this defensive structure as the expression of the only hope that remains: "If I cannot get what I want by hook, I get it by crook." Once a child embarks on that route, however, this psychic solution will then of course create a life of its own: a life based on secrecy, distrust, fear, and one which precludes any possibility for genuine intimacy. In fact, it may put such person in a position where even getting therapeutic help becomes impossible because it is seen as endangering the secrets (Liz's case history is an example).

Mood disorders run in families. They do so for several reasons. One is genetic predisposition. However, even without a biological vulnerability, children of depressed parents are at a considerably higher risk for depression than children of nondepressed parents. According to extensive field studies by Myrna Weissman (1989) the increase in risk is threefold. Systematic observation of the interaction between depressed parents and their children readily explains why. Depression, particularly when it is severe, interferes with the adult's capacity for empathy and attunement. The depressed parent, teacher, therapist, or spouse has to devote an inordinate amount of time and attention to the simple task of just getting out of bed in the morning and then through all the tasks of the day without being engulfed by despair. If psychomotor retardation is part of the clinical picture, just feeding a baby can seem a monumental task. Sensitivity to noise and visual stimuli is pronounced, which means that a rambunctious toddler is experienced as a form of divine punishment. Yadke-Yarrow (1988) who observed pairs of depressed mothers and their children, found that: (1) Depressed mothers were more likely to back off when they met resistance from their children while trying to control them. These mothers appeared uncertain and helpless, a typical symptom of depression; (2) Depressed mothers were less able to compromise in disagreements with their children and they often confused their children's normal attempts at independence with "breaking the rules"; (3) While making and eating lunch the depressed mothers spoke less frequently than the controls; and (4) When the depressed mothers did speak with their children, they made more negative comments than did other mothers. In general, unipolar depression makes people more self-centered, withdrawn, weepy, irritable, short-tempered, or, alternately, clinging or rejecting, inattentive, indecisive, incapable of experiencing or expressing joy, and hopeless. All of these symptoms impair the capacity for empathy and attunement with the feelings and the needs of another person. For example, the mother who returned from a three-month hospital stay, where she recovered from a postpartum depression, discovered to her great dismay that her baby, now three months old, responded to her with the warmth of a porcupine. It recoiled from her touch, rarely met her eyes, and was generally unresponsive. It never occurred to her that what the baby exhibited, behaviorally, were all the signs and symptoms of an abandonment depression. She experienced her child as rejecting *her*, and she responded with hurt and anger, about as absolute a mother-child mismatch as one can imagine.

The relationship between the bipolar parent and his or her child is even more damaging and more complex. Interpersonally the bipolar parent resembles the alcoholic parent in that the main characteristic of their reactions to their offspring is unpredictability in terms of mood, cognition, and availability. The environment that such a parent generates puts the child through cycles of omnipotence and impotence, grandiosity and shame, elation and depression, love and hate. The manic patient at the height of the manic phase creates an atmosphere which typically is characterized by the urgency and insistence of a narcissistically hungry infant, one lacking in the necessary external care and vehemently demanding the much needed emotional supplies. The profound object hunger that is displayed has little to do with the qualities or characteristics of the human object itself; rather, it pertains to the narcissistic usage that the object may have at any particular moment. The child, then, may well be seduced into wanting to be a jewel in mother's crown, even though experience has taught the child that soon it will become a thorn in mother's side, and that eventually it will vanish from mother's sight altogether. In this way the parent inappropriately stimulates the child's grandiosity only to thoroughly deflate it at a later point, without the child having any sense of a causal relationship in this sequence of events. The other common interactive pattern between the bipolar parent and the child is that during the manic phase the child becomes the parent's magical little helper, even protector. While in the course of the depressed phase the parent has to be cheered up, consoled, and coaxed into living, during the manic stretch the parent must be pacified, fed, and looked after, and the child is hoping that in that way it partakes in the parent's omnipotence. Also, the child must learn how to respond to the extreme vulnerability of the manic parent to even the slightest or most minimal narcissistic injuries. It must become extraordinarily diplomatic to avoid inflicting such slights, lest it become the object of the parent's wrath. During the depressive phase the child feels abandoned, shut out, is made to feel as if it were the "cause" of all the parent's misery. Depending on the severity of the bipolar disorder in the parent, she or he may well be considered to be quite handicapped in their role as parent.

In fact, E. James Anthony feels: "As a parent, the manic-depressive is loaded with damaging deficiencies: he takes but refuses to give; he has little awareness of others as people but only as stereotypes and consequently has little capacity to empathize with them; he shows minimal respect for reality and is always ready to substitute magical manipulation for realistic reaction and interaction. The combination of infantile dependency, manipulativeness, exploitation, shallowness, insensibility to give anything of himself and the very extroverted approach to reality renders the manic-depressive unfit for the complex task of parenthood and puts his children at risk for some form of depression at all stages of their development" (1985, p. 314).

This is a harsh judgment indeed, with little hope for the unfortunate children raised by such parents. The concordance rate for bipolar disorder in families with a bipolar parent appears to substantiate that contention. However, it does *not* explain what happens to the children of such parents who do *not* develop the disorder, who grow up relatively unscathed. Studies of such children have shown several things. First of all, they typically have had access to alternate caretakers, such as other family members, grandparents, siblings, neighbors, teachers, pets, or maids. Secondly, disturbed parents tend to select one child as the main target for the expression of their pathology. The ones not serving that function, comparatively speaking, merely suffer from "benign neglect." Furthermore, siblings can be astonishingly protective of each other, showing signs of compassion, empathy, and consolation as early as at the age of two. Finally, the "resilient child," according to Radke-Yarrow, is unusually talented in seeking substitute caretakers; they tend to have "winning smiles," are attractive and engaging, and they manage to elicit the absolute maximum of emotional supply, tapping each and every last resource that such families have to offer.

Of the psychosocial factors predisposing children to depression, parental depression ranks quite high. However, other variables have also been identified. In terms of parental psychopathology, narcissistic disturbances stand out, as do substance abuse, alcoholism, and drug addiction, prolonged illness on the part of one or both parents, prolonged separations without adequate caretakers, extreme poverty or deprivation, early losses due to death of parents, grandparents, siblings, or pets; in other words, any chaotic conditions that disrupt the continuity of the affective bonds and significantly interfere with the orderly unfolding of the natural endowment of a particular infant.

Additionally, certain personality traits, such as shyness or introversion, play a dual role in the etiology of depression. First of all, they are to some degree genetically determined. For a child raised in a stable family or in a rural or small-town environment, this trait may cause no problems. That same child, raised in a single-parent household in an urban setting, attending an overcrowded school system and subjected to repeated geographic moves in the course of growing up, could find that same shyness quite a handicap in developing a social support system to help weather developmental crises. Alternatively, a depressed child or adult, already only too inclined to isolate itself due to its depressed mood, will be unlikely to utilize the depression-free periods to build these support systems and to actually utilize them when depression sets in. Introversion and depression thus can easily create a vicious cycle where the victim can honestly say, "I would like to help myself by going out more often, but I truly have no friends."

Finally, since social isolation plays such a pivotal role in the etiology of depression, the type of character-armor—the particular flavor of a person's interactive style—also plays a major role: some character-pathology simply is more off-putting than others. For example, in Kohut's distinction in pathological narcissism, characterized by what he calls a "horizontal split," a person presents to the world a passive, unassuming, slightly dejected self, while the grandiosity is firmly repressed. The person who exhibits what Kohut refers to as a "vertical split," shows the world the haughty, arrogant, contemptuous "being better than anybody else" self, with the obverse, namely the insecure empty self, firmly repressed. Such people, unless they are born royalty, may have followers but very few friends. If too much of their disdain for humanity shows, they live their lives in splendid isolation.

Finally, as I discussed in the chapter on biology, some specific physiological disturbances such as hormonal and neurotransmitter imbalances may precipitate a depressive episode or, rather, they often constitute the proverbial straw that breaks the camel's back. Taken together, some or all of the variables listed here in their interaction and in response to real-life events contribute to what has been called "the final common pathway." Real and stressful life events may be just that, stressful, but they need not be depressing in their effect, as for example that rite of passage of completing a college education or a Ph.D. dissertation (an entrance event), unless the new Ph.D. is focused primarily on the loss of the role of student, with all the caretaking privileges that may entail. Typically, however, the events that precipitate depression are genuine exit events such as divorce, retirement, or the death of a loved one. They spell loss of either human or nonhuman objects, relationships, status, goals, body image, self-concept, or identity. While the role of *acute* stress in the etiology of depression has been known and studied for a long time, recent research has also shown that the accumulative effect of low-level, chronic, and unpredictable stress is at least as, if not more, decisive in pushing the organism towards that final common pathway we call depression. This probably explains the inordinately high incidence of depression among poor and working-class women with small children who are single heads of households.

We can now return to the case material presented in Chapter two in order to examine whether and how the interrelationship between these five variables contributed to the development of a depression among those specific individuals. First of all, it is important to point out that tracing the history of what constitutes the final common pathway usually does not show a linear progression of an accumulation of debilitating and demoralizing factors which, taken together, ran a person down. To the contrary, the years preceding a breakdown may reveal a heroic tale of resilience and courage.

Peter, a gifted musician, is an example of this. When at the age of 70 he and his wife Ruth retired to Florida they saw it as the culmination of many happy years they had spent together; they looked forward to their "golden years." However, within a few months of their move south, Ruth suddenly died from a viral infection. Peter, after a period of intense mourning, soon befriended a recent widow and for the next several years it seemed that they would be a happy couple. However, Peter's new girlfriend, who had assumed that Peter was much wealthier than he said he was, grew restless, and began to look for another spouse. When she found one, she abruptly left Peter. Peter himself, who had had no chance to make friends of his own, prior to Ruth's death, and who had been welcomed into the circle of friends of his lady friend, suddenly found himself all alone, with music as his sole consolation. He vaguely sensed that a depression was waiting for him. As a consequence, he looked around for a project to occupy him, preferably one which addressed his grief and his loneliness at the same time. He found it in the German art-song, whose texts are full of death, dying, grief, tears, lost loves, dead or dying children. All existing translations into English happen to be extremely poor. Peter took the songs most commonly performed and he began the job of translation. For some of them, mostly Schubert lieder, he also transcribed the piano score for the violin. He had a new and all-consuming passion and, except for an occasional blue day, he did well emotionally. Then Peter's ancient cat began to ail and, finally, she died. Peter became frightened by the increasing intensity of what he considered to be his "blue days." Although, there were more losses, worst of all, in the condominium where he lived, he acquired a new neighbor, a "country-western" fan who was quite deaf and most inconsiderate. Peter kept bouncing back, redoubling his efforts on his "project." His blood pressure kept rising and his medication for hypertension was changed. His battle with depression grew worse. Finally, Peter, who had been under the impression that his manuscript had been accepted for publication, learned that, due to some changes in the tax laws, his publisher had decided to eliminate all projects that did not have a short but lucrative shelf-life. Peter's book was one of those that were scratched from the list. Peter persisted; he resubmitted his manuscript to several different publishing houses, was rejected, and tried again. Eventually, eight years after Ruth's death, Peter took an overdose of barbiturates; but he survived. The surprising aspect of this story is *not* that Peter became suicidally depressed, but the many different ways which this resilient German-Jewish expatriate found to creatively counteract an impending breakdown.

1. If we examine the "clinical infant" in our case histories, Martha, Mary, Liz, and Bernie, we know that in the families of the first three there existed unipolar and bipolar depression: Martha's mother and Mary and Liz's fathers. It does not seem too farfetched to suspect that Bernie's parents probably suffered from low-level depression as well, during their lives in the States. What we do know is that three out of four of these patients were born genetically at risk. How much at risk we cannot say, only at some risk.

2. As to developmental events: Martha's upbringing was left to a large extent to maids, while her mother saw her role essentially as her husband's helpmate and as that of a semi-professional musician. While the concept of the "child-centered household" was not yet invented, that particular household was unique even by the standards of that time, in that family life paled in importance compared to that of the "salon" aspect socially and academically. It was a gathering place for intellectuals, where children were seldom seen and hardly ever heard, unless they had something brilliant to say, hardly a likely proposition for a toddler. In that particular view of the verbal role of children we have a clear case of "selective attunement," one to which the child learns to also filter its verbal productions in such a way that they respond to the particular interest of the parents.

By the time Mary was born, the family unit was already beginning to seriously disintegrate. The two oldest siblings were in their teens and rarely home, and Mary's father's work history had become sufficiently erratic to require serious belt-tightening. Soon, her mother had to take over the role of the breadwinner. Her father's drinking began to rock the family equilibrium in that he became the "identified child or patient," *the* problem, the center around which everything revolved. Mary's mother was primarily concerned with the problem of maintaining a facade of respectability, being far too self-involved to be able to be properly attuned to the needs of her younger children. Moreover, she looked more and more to Mary as a helpmate in dealing with her querulous husband. Here we have an instance where clearly it was the job of the child to be maximally attuned to needs of the parents, instead of the other way around. That kind of role reversal is quite common among dysfunctional families.

Liz's family life was very similar in the way it functioned. Additionally, the adoption of two orphans when the two youngest ones were still quite young spelled inexplicable losses that the children could not understand. They were asked to stand back in terms of access to emotional and financial resources, clothes, beds, space, and specialness. Natural sibling rivalry was undercut by the accusation of "selfishness," lack of Christian charity, and shabby greed. This strange family arrangement certainly contributed to Liz's permanent sense of being misunderstood, falsely accused, suspected of having ulterior motives, being untrustworthy and dishonest. She developed a chronic case of distrust, one which, tragically, she then substantiated in the eyes of the world with her very actions.

Bernie, being separated from his parents as a toddler, had to deal with two major losses: loss of parents and loss of country, with its familiar language. After the war he was again uprooted, separated from his foster parents, another familiar place, and then had to get reacquainted with his own parents whom he had thought he had lost. Then he had to live in a country even stranger than the one before. Bernie's challenge as a small child was to discern what kinds of actions on his part would earn or elicit caretaking behavior on the part of adults who were not his parents and therefore not obligated to look after him. He had to be precocious in his ability to discern the needs of others. Ultimately, he must have concluded, the best solution would be for him to become as self-sufficient as possible and to *never* again be in a position of true need.

3. Regarding psychological stresses: The years preceding Martha's depression were punctuated by losses—husband, children, self-image, physical integrity (i.e., health and beauty, social network and role), in other words, all the attributes that had previously defined her as a person and had given her social status, and all the functions that had defined her and supplied her with a purpose in life, had vanished and could not yet be replaced.

The first time Mary came close to having a breakdown was after her father died. She escaped it by resorting to what in criminal circles is known as "taking the geographic." She moved across the country, and lived the life of a vagabond. During that time of being constantly on the move, her mania eventually dissipated. Since she also did not work at all then, she could move entirely at her own pace, without the stress of time pressure or other obligations, or performance anxiety. The second time around, it was very different. A considerable variety of different stress factors, taken together, pushed her over the edge and into a manic-depressive breakdown. She had been working very hard in her psychotherapy; she seriously dealt with her professional aspiration and with what her vocational life might hold for her. For reasons that are still not entirely clear, neither parent had paid any attention to Mary's education past high school. It was simply assumed that attending nursing school would be sufficient, even though almost everybody else in her family had graduated from college. Now, as an adult, Mary not only went to college, she had a love affair with learning; nothing but straight A's would do. In terms of intelligence and academic accomplishment, Mary's father, for no reason at all, had mocked her cruelly, clearly projecting his own sense of shame onto his daughter. Consequently, for every A that Mary received, she had to pay with terror attacks before each exam and term paper. She overprepared continuously and, even though this was an extremely positive development for her, it cost her dearly in terms of stress, which included the stress of therapeutic work. The actual loss of her aunt, the family member she had been closest to, together with her mother's surgery for breast cancer, changed Mary's life dramatically. First of all, these two women were the only family members Mary had spoken to in over five years. Secondly, she became the sole caretaker of her aunt, who, in addition to general ill health and old age also suffered from Alzheimer's disease. Mary finally had to put her into a nursing home where she was the only member of that family who not only came to visit, but who did so almost daily. Though Mary's mother recovered remarkably well from surgery, the event nevertheless signaled to Mary the fact that soon she would be all alone in the world—a frightening prospect for a person with so few human ties.

Liz's first two breakdowns had probably been triggered by two developmental events, one of which was also hormonal. Leaving home and starting vocational school is clearly a "passage" event, a major role transition from childhood into adult life. Judging by the medication she was given both times, she was probably diagnosed as being either what today would be called a "borderline structure" or a schizophrenic. Her remarkably fast recovery, in spite of this inappropriate treatment, is quite a powerful testimony to her strength and her survival skills. Her second breakdown, a postpartum psychosis, was a much more complex event. While, temporarily, at least, the second child most likely solidified her marriage, it also must have been extremely stressful, given the fact that she had come to pretty much despise her blue-collar spouse. To complicate things further, given her homosexual orientation, she experienced the "straight" marriage as prison, one which was about to suffocate her. Again, her quick recovery, in spite of a medication that was inappropriate, i.e., without the Lithium she probably needed desperately, is quite astonishing. Nevertheless, she must have known on some level that her life was becoming increasingly unsafe, given her vulnerabilities, lack of effective treatment, and stressful life. I suspect that on some level she sensed that she might not always be this lucky and this strong, that she might not always be able to pull herself up by her own bootstraps. In that sense, wisely, she took flight, though that meant leaving a husband, a home, and two children. From then on, her love life and particularly her relationships with nine different therapists over the course of the next 15 years added to her already quite tumultuous existence. It reinforced her mood swings, and thus her affective life was a continuous emotional roller-coaster. The quality of her relationships with lovers and that with her therapists seems to have been very similar. Those were intense sadomasochistic involvements which eventually culminated in an intense emotional explosion followed by separation. Her interpersonal life itself was bipolar in its dramatic style.

Bernie had been groomed for the role of family ambassador to a hostile world; his becoming a university professor would have redeemed them all. While he pursued this goal with admirable determination until he received his Ph.D. degree, another part of him was equally determined to undermine this pursuit: he pseudo-innocently disregarded the "publish or perish" doctrine which governs academia. Denying Bernie a tenured position was an entirely predictable course of action on the part of the college where he taught. What had been disappointed, then, was not a realistic expectation, but an unconscious belief in magic, the hope that just once in his life just "being" could be rewarded. When this did not happen, Bernie stopped playing with a full deck. In a way, his life in his Village studio apartment and his neighborhood bars was as narrowly circumscribed as his parents' living room had been.

For almost the next 20 years nothing was allowed to disturb his peace and to disrupt his precarious equilibrium, until the age of 47. Then his self-esteem suffered two serious blows, one from his girlfriend and one from the editor he so admired. He was challenged to look at his life, to examine it, and he could not bear to see what he saw. He took no action. Instead he tried to kill his pain with vodka. It was as if he were trying to stop his awakening from almost two decades of hibernation. He had never had a stable home, a secure sense of belonging, or a firm sense of self. What he had built for himself was a fragile shelter to protect him from an all-pervasive sense of homelessness and alienation. It was as if he had never really left Ellis Island, hardly a surprising development, since nothing in his early life had equipped him to make himself at home in this world, and to trust that it would not disappoint him again.

3. Physiological stresses: In Martha's case there were a considerable number of physiological variables that contributed to her depression on a biological level. Menopause, arthritis, pancreatitis, besides making life miserable in general, all affect the hormonal equilibrium, and consequently, neurotransmitter activity. While men do not experience the equivalent of menopause, with age they too nevertheless go through hormonal changes that are not too dissimilar. Turning 50 years of age, from a neurohormonal point of view, then, is a stressful event, one which most likely contributed to Bernie's vulnerability. Also, his history of drinking, and three years of alcoholic drinking patterns undoubtedly did little to protect him from depression.

Liz had suffered from a postpartum psychosis—also to a considerable degree a hormonal event. Throughout her adult life she suffered from PMS (premenstrual syndrome). At the time when her "tailspins" became severe enough to require medication, even in her evaluation, she was approaching menopause.

Mary was in her late 30s when she had her breakdown, and one could argue that she was too young for even the precursors of menopause. However, a series of endocrine tests clearly showed that she had undergone marked hormonal changes which were identical with those that are typical of premenopausal women. To sort out cause and effect with respect to the progression of bipolar disorder and sex hormones is not possible because neuroleptics affect the menstrual cycle and several hormonal mechanisms and vice versa. At this point, we simply don't know enough.

4 and 5. Personality traits and character pathology: Evaluating the effect of personality traits and character pathology on the etiology, obviously, is very much a chicken/egg problem. While

shyness and introversion are to some extent inborn features, that does not mean that they could not be counteracted by remedial efforts on the part of the parents. However, in the typical run of events, shy children grow into shy adults. Nobody expects them to take leadership positions; they are natural and often valued followers and some of them become loners. Of equal importance, in this context, is the acquisition of social skills, knowing how to interact with other people, even if it is only on a superficial level. A more solitary life in and of itself need not be a hardship—but being unable to relate to others, feeling left out, involuntarily isolated, is injurious and leads to depression. Social skills, then, have a triple function: (1) They may protect a person from sliding into a depression in the first place; (2) they influence the depth and the duration of a depression; and (3) they are an indispensable part of the recovery. In a more general vein, since social support systems seem to be one of the most important variables in determining the onset, duration, and recovery rate, at least of unipolar depression, any personality trait, as well as any type of character pathology, that interferes with a person's ability to form or maintain close human ties is an essential ingredient as antecedent as well as determinant of the course of a depression.

Martha, for example, hardly lacked social skills, but she was basically a very reserved person with a forbidding exterior which bordered on being haughty and snobbish. All her married life she never had to take any initiative when it came to meeting new people and to maintaining relationships with old friends. On the contrary, it was her job to discourage Rob's gregariousness, to make sure there was some time when the house was not full of people. Thus, as a part of a marital team there was never a problem having enough people available. But once she was alone, she felt desperately lonely. Her enormous pride did not permit her to seek out people, to appear needy, or to mix with people she did not consider to be her intellectual equals. The line between being discriminating and being dismissive can be a thin one indeed; Martha clearly erred on the side of being overly critical, which contributed to her social isolation and thus rendered her more vulnerable to depression.

Bernie, too was at ease socially. He knew how to engage people from all walks of life and he was an excellent listener. However, he was basically shy and introverted. He kept his inner life, the dreams of glory as well as his hurts and disappointments, pretty much to himself, as did Martha. His relationships with people lacked depth and intimacy. When he fell apart, he did so without anybody noticing. His friends had thoughts about his drinking habits, but nobody was at all aware that Bernie was in serious and desperate emotional trouble. The explanatory framework within which his friends could adequately fit his changed behavior was: "Again, Bernie had one too many." It did not occur to anyone to investigate what its real meaning might be. In that way, Bernie kept screaming for help without anybody hearing him. Unconsciously, he kept hoping that someone would take notice before he took the drastic step of publicly overdosing. Once he was sober, Bernie came to the painful realization that too many of his "friends" were, essentially, "drinking buddies." He had to start making real friends.

Mary had grown up in a family that had already isolated itself from the world in order to hide its many secrets and in order to protect the family pathology from the outside world. As a consequence, all that Mary learned were the manners of a proper lady. She knew how to play the role of an adoring audience, how to be a faithful helpmate of whoever happened to ask her, and how to be a perfect listener to other people's troubles. What she did not learn at all was how to have a friendship that is based on intimacy, equality, respect for differences of opinion, personal style, or interests, as well as tolerance and separateness. Not knowing the difference between symbiosis and love, Mary kept hoping for a merger with an omnipotent, omniscient lover, and she was prepared for any interpersonal sacrifice that such a relationship would demand from her. In reality, Mary had very few friends, and she was desperately lonely. Furthermore, given her vulnerabilities, Mary's dream was of course also her most frightening nightmare, namely to be devoured by another person. In that sense, Mary's isolation was wise and appropriate. What she had yet to learn about was the safe space between isolation and engulfment.

Liz, interpersonally, had perhaps the most complex and intractable problems. She had *not* been taught how to be a lady, or even the most rudimentary display of middle-class manners. What she had at her disposal was an assemblage of pieces of interpersonal relating, a patchwork quilt, really, that ranged from the most abrasive to the exquisitely intuitive. When it came to discerning what another human being might want as the kind of gift only a fairy godmother could imagine and procure, Liz was an utter genius. She spared neither time nor effort in crafting the most extraordinary gifts. They never represented her *own* interests or style; they were truly geared to the world of the other person. On occasion she could also produce a rational colleague self that met the other on the most understanding level. Unfortunately, the abusive end of the behavioral spectrum was such that no friendship could possibly endure the onslaught of the corrosive and explosive quality of her words. From her father she had learned gutter language that would have made the proverbial sailor blush. Furthermore, feminism, radical lesbianism, and psychoanalysis had supplied her with additional ingredients for motivational attributions, sufficient to mortally wound just about anybody who, in a flash of rage, she chose to annihilate. Being a masterful manipulator, she was also an accomplished provocateur. In order to vent her pent-up rage, she typically felt it necessary to first become that person's "victim." At this art she was an expert. It took her hardly any time or effort to goad the unsuspecting victim into some response that she would then claim "wounded her terribly." But once she had gotten the desired response, she then felt free to retaliate, pulling out all the stops. In that way she resembled a small child, who is flinging its dolls around, totally oblivious of its effect on the dolls.

Liz, being what clinically is called a "borderline personality," one whose major defensive mode is "splitting," did not experience the discontinuity in her relationship with people as at all unusual. It seemed perfectly natural to her that she should detest all her previous lovers and psychotherapists, since they had betrayed her; they were human vermin and she was lucky to be rid of them. She truly had no inkling of her own role as the agent provocateur. To acquire insight into her own actions was particularly difficult for Liz because of her extreme vulnerability to criticism and therefore, shame. Where other people can simply goof, her goofs were always of such major proportions that they qualified as unforgivable failings, even sins. There was no room for ordinary mistakes because there was no room for anything that was not either "all good" or "all bad," all black or all white. In other words, the gray shades that characterize ordinary human beings did not exist in her world. Finally, as will be shown later, Liz's psychopathy eventually proved to be her biggest handicap. The intricate network of circumvented or ignored financial and legal obligations made it extremely difficult to resurface and to join the law-abiding, tax-paying, professional middle-class.

The final common pathway then, constitutes the interactive and/or cumulative effect of at least five groups of variables. To try to quantify them in terms of their relative weight and importance would be a futile enterprise, given our still limited knowledge. It is of course always tempting to speculate in each instance what might have happened if—if, for example, Rob had died only five years later than he did; if Liz had been born into the professional middle class; if Mary had joined a convent, and if Bernie had taught in a private boarding school. Alternatively, we can think about how much worse things might have been had Martha been a refugee, if Mary had been less attractive, if Liz had been less articulate and intelligent. All are intriguing questions. None of them have answers.

On the other hand, what we are beginning to understand a little better, is how the talking cure can help. Perhaps, as we understand these relationships even better, we will get some sense of the relative weight of the variables under discussion.

How Psychotherapy Heals

Psychotherapy is basically the art of teaching an old dog new tricks. It can consist of any type of intervention aimed at disrupting, changing, or rechanneling a learned behavior or behavioral sequence. One of the most fascinating experiments aimed at preventing an *anticipated* outcome of a behavioral sequence was conducted in England by John Bowlby and his associates. The research team identified young couples where one or both spouses had been abused as children and where the wife had just become pregnant for the first time. They rightly assumed that these unborn children were at risk for abuse. Bowlby then assembled a group of middle-aged couples, untrained volunteers, and assigned one set of volunteers to each of these young couples. The concept underlying this assignment was to "mother the mother." All that was asked of these sets of foster grandparents was to drop in several times a week, share a cup of coffee, shoot the breeze, listen to the mother, maybe mind the baby for an hour, or help the young woman go shopping. But mostly their purpose was to lend an ear, or a shoulder, to be there, rather than to help with the actual work. In all the years that this program has been in operation there has not been *one case* of child abuse, when on the basis of statistical probability alone, there should have been several. This is psychotherapy in its most rudimentary form. Abuse, certainly, had been a behavioral possibility for these parents who had been on the receiving end of that particular interactive emotional short circuit that transducts or translates hurt and frustration into rage and physical violence. Obviously they also knew other ways of responding to these same feelings, namely to alleviate the baby's distress, not to interpret its crying as a judgment or an indictment of their ability to mother, and they acquired the capacity to simply walk away from the stress, etc. As it turned out, these mothers chose over and over again to execute benign resolutions to the demands made by their children; not once did they break through the sound barrier where frustration turns into aggression towards the frustrating object.

Psychotherapy, as it is defined by the dictionary, implies intervention or an attempt to cure: "the psychological treatment of mental, emotional, and nervous disorders." Treatment, then, presupposes the existence of a pathological condition. Even though the mothers in Bowlby's group had not yet manifested any disorder, I would still argue that what took place qualifies in a small way as treatment because one particular potential out of several that could have been possible never unfolded, while several others were repeatedly exercised and reinforced. Basic learning theory suggests that this development decreases the probability that the violent option will be exercised in the future due to the fact that under those specific circumstances, with foster grandparents available, those young women experienced mothering as a manageable, even pleasant and rewarding task. In addition, these mothers had the repeated experience that verbalizing one's frustrations to another adult is likely to have beneficial results. Equally important, they learned that they can be both the subject and the object of soothing and comforting.

In this particular context, psychotherapy is seemingly reduced to a simple learning process; except that there is nothing "simple" about the mechanisms that are at work. The introduction to this book mentions Kandel's famous experiment with the sea snail *Aplysia Californica*. What makes this experiment so important in the history of neurobiology *and psychotherapy,* is the fact that it showed for the first time that experience can result in long-lasting neurological changes. Specifically, it demonstrated that in response to repeated tapping of the spout of this animal, the neurons involved, which number less than 100, released fewer neurotransmitters into the synapses than before over-stimulation, thus changing the organism's neurological signal to withdraw the gill. This process is called habituation. Its obverse, namely sensitization, accomplishes the opposite. Increased amounts of neurotransmitter amplify a message. In other words: *Cells themselves can learn and remember!*

It was Kandel himself who, in 1979, made the connection between the neuronal changes in the gill-withdrawing system of the sea snails and the process of psychotherapy.

> When I speak to someone and he or she listens to me, we can not only make eye contact and voice contact, but the action of the neuronal machinery in my brain is having a direct and, I hope, long-lasting effect on the neuronal machinery in his or her brain, and vice versa. Indeed, I would argue that it is only insofar as our words produce changes in each other's brains that psycho-therapeutic intervention produces changes in patients' minds. (p.1037)

But how do we connect the simple reflex of the *Aplysia* with the more complex behavioral sets?

First of all, there are no fundamental functional or bio-chemical differences between the nerve cells, the neurotransmit-ters, and synapses of man and those of that snail. The ability to store information as memory is a universal function of all ner-vous systems, however primitive. All animals possess the ability for elementary forms of learning, and all of these forms of learn-ing give rise to both long-term and short-term memory. Since behavior is a complex reflection of nerve cell activity, it should not be surprising that the behavior of man has at least some elementary features in common with that of the *Aplysia*. Many of the basic mechanisms found in simple systems are apt to be utilized in modular fashion by higher forms of life.

What is more, some of the latest findings about gene ex-pression in long-term memory have important implications for psychotherapy. To appreciate their import we have to first understand how cells do what they do, once they are part of an organ. Each cell in the body contains all the genes present in every other cell. (There are two exceptions, but they are not of relevance in this context.) In humans that amounts to somewhere between 100,000 and 1 million genes. What makes a brain cell act like a brain cell, as distinguished from, for example, a stomach cell, is the cell's ability to shut off the activity of certain genes while letting others be expressed. As a result, in any given cell there are many genes that are not transcribed, only some of them are competent and available for transcription. In psychiatric disorders that are primarily genetically determined, such as schizophrenia and bipolar depression, due to a gene mutation, we find an alteration in the *structure* of genes. Neurosis, acquired by learning, and therefore amenable to psychotherapeutic intervention, in contrast, involves alterations in the structure and function of synapses by producing alterations in the regulation of gene *expression*. Obviously, patients suffering from psychiatric disorders which are caused by inherited alterations in gene structure, may also exhibit a set of secondary disturbances in environmentally acquired gene expression. According to Kandel, as the resolution of modern brain-imaging techniques increases, it appears likely that these alterations could be measured. That means that these techniques could be used not only for diagnostic purposes, but they would also constitute a tool for measuring the outcome of psychotherapy in terms of changes in gene expression.

In addition, neuronal changes are not restricted to neurotransmitters' activity alone. For example, in a series of experiments conducted at Yale, rat pups were raised in three different environments: one was what the investigators called the "enriched environment," full of toys and objects that happen to be of great interest to rats; the second was a normal environment; the third was one where the rats were kept in small cages within the larger enriched environment—i.e., the rats in these cages could watch the rats in the enriched environment at play, but they themselves could not participate. I am tempted to call this group the "television group" or the "couch potatoes." At the end of this experiment the brains of all three groups were examined under the microscope. It turned out that the rats in the enriched environment had grown additional dendrites on their brains, meaning in addition to the ones they were born with, while the rats in the normal environment and the couch potatoes showed no changes. The first group's active involvement with problem solving and coming to grips with the environment had actually increased the complexity of their neuronal machinery. Learning had, so to speak, literally swelled their heads. What is even more intriguing is the fact that when these experiments were repeated with adult rats the results were identical (Rosenzweig, 1972).

Given what we already know about the psychobiological mechanisms operating in rats, it seems entirely justified to extrapolate from these findings the appropriate lessons for humans, i.e., various sets of hypotheses applicable to the higher level of complexity found in humans. John L. Haracs (1984), who refers to the process of experience-induced brain changes as neural plasticity, has argued that findings such as those just mentioned are entirely compatible with some of the basic tenets of psychoanalytic metapsychology (or any school of psychotherapy, I might add). For example, if we take the psychoanalytic concept of fixation and look at it from this perspective we can see the following: Neural plasticity here denotes the modulation of transmission efficacy (i.e., electrophysiological efficacy of existing synapses, as well as the formation or degeneration of synapses). Thus, theoretically, the brain can make structural and functional adaptations to accommodate impinging stimuli, i.e., experiences originating in the environment. Increased usage of specific neural pathways leads to increased structural and functional developments of those pathways, while inactive pathways may lose synapses or efficiency. Among the most dramatic findings in this area are the studies of monkeys that were raised in social isolation (Sonnier, 1981). These animals developed a variety of abnormal behaviors, including self-clasping and -biting, retarded motor activity, avoidance of social contact, fearfulness, and a lack of appropriate sexual behavior patterns. Microscopic examination of the brains of these monkeys at age six to eight months revealed dendritic branching deficits in the cells of the cerebral and cerebellar cortices, reflecting an altered synaptic organization. Since behaviorally these monkeys resemble human infants with severe developmental disturbances, such as autism, it seems reasonable to assume that these childhood disorders may correspond to dendritic deficiencies and changes in synaptic organization. The abnormal neural structures were particularly pronounced in the supplementary motor area (SMA) which is responsible for the programming of voluntary motor behavior in higher primates. Controlled movements are vital components of social behavior, of purposeful social interactions.

While stereotypic behaviors, such as rocking, are developmental stages in monkey and man alike, they increasingly are replaced with controlled behavioral responses. Among the isolated monkeys, that shift did not occur; more accurately, the proportion of stereotypic to refined motor skills in these deprived animals remained skewed. Biologically, then, what can be seen is a developmental arrest, a "fixation" at a lower level of branching complexity. Thus the physiological arrest and the psychological fixation may be each other's psychobiological counterparts, since the SMA probably contributes to the generation of socially related motor behaviors.

Our understanding of the physiological basis for long-term memory points in a similar direction. Experiments with repetitive electrostimulation have shown that even a single application of that kind of stimulus can have a lasting impact on neuronal pathways by enhancing them selectively, i.e., by increasing the amount of neurotransmitter released or by sensitization of the postsynaptic receptor membrane. This phenomenon, known as long-term potentiation (LTP), is frequently discussed as the experimental model of long-term memory because the parameters employed resemble the natural firing patterns of neurons in behaving animals. Such potentiation of transmission has been observed during the behavioral conditioning of mice and rabbits. In cats the transmission efficiencies of limbic pathways were found to vary systematically with feline personality characteristics such as defensive vs. aggressive response patterns. It seems that aggressive cats have naturally enhanced transmission efficiencies in pathways that facilitate aggression.

Hypothetically, if we apply these considerations to Bowlby's experiment, we know that the young parents in his study had clear memories of being hit as a result of another person's frustration. The reverse process, namely one's own frustration resulting in physical injury of one's own child had not yet taken place: the pathway from A–Z was already established, while the pathway Z–A was merely a potential. The new experience of being mothered while in the process of mothering—or preceding the mothering behavior—derailed the behavior potential by creating new pathways in the form of behavioral alternatives to violence by either inhibiting aggression or by making the alternatives more pleasurable or plausible, or both.

Unlike other cells, the 10 to 100 billion neurons that we are born with do not regenerate if destroyed. However, existing neurons can become more complex in structure, function, and chemical composition. They can grow new connections, modify old ones in a variety of ways, including changes in shape of dendritic thorns and the size and structure of synapses. Electrical stimulation can expose new receptor molecules and clusters of newly exposed receptors can migrate and form the receiving ends of entirely new synapses and circuits (sprouting). Neurons can also increase their production of key enzymes which are involved in the production and the breakdown of neurotransmitter molecules. Glands, in contrast, including those that secrete behaviorally active molecules, can become larger and smaller in response to use and, unlike neurons, they have the potential for producing new cells by cell division.

Theoretically, one can think of psychosis in humans as a reactivation of archaic infantile neural pathways (Post, 1977).

Repetitive stressful experiences in childhood, then, may potentiate genetically more or less vulnerable limbic catecholaminergic pathways and thereby predispose the individual to future psychopathology. Stressful events in later life might trigger a psychotic episode by reactivating the potentiated pathways, while the same stresses can be experienced by someone who is not so predisposed as merely stressful—even harmless. Reactivation, or mobilization of other pathways, fits the clinical picture of some patients much better than constructs such as regression. Clinical observations tend to be notoriously unreliable, in that we clinicians tend to see what we are looking for, or what we expect on the basis of theory. However, even to the untrained eye, there appears to be a remarkable difference between the suddenness of the cognitive-affective switches of, say, a rapidly cycling bipolar patient and the gradual regression observed in a different kind of patient. In the case of the bipolar phenomenon, there is simply no mistaking the fact that something quite abrupt and extraordinary is happening in front of our eyes. The concept of regression implies a continuous moving back in time and space comparable to the workings of a zoom lens; the visual image that comes to mind with the bipolar patient is rather that of a number of model train tracks, where the train might capriciously jump back and forth between different tracks at any of a number of random switching stations, or at no obvious intersection at all. The same randomness seems to characterize the cognitive circuits traveled by a bipolar patient's trains of thought. Furthermore, the clusters of thoughts and corresponding feelings, like the fixed tracks and small dead scenery of a toy train table, tend to be extremely repetitive and stereotypical for each patient or individual. There are rarely any new data or associations. Once the leap has been made to, say, the "victimization" track, the incidents supporting this position are rattled off like train stations or the immutable exits on an expressway, until the next extreme leap is made. What is so remarkable in such cases is the degree to which affective coloration and trains of thought are welded together.

Reiser (1984), who has proposed that the major psychoses could be conceptualized as stress disorders with the brain as the target organ—a claim that is both brilliant and provocative— uses a similar analogy in his description of CNS circuits, both normal and pathogenic. He suggests we imagine a TV studio with a live drama with many cameras recording the same scene from different angles, perspectives, and distances. The film director, scanning the monitor constantly, has to make choices as to which of the multiple versions to present to the audience. He can also accomplish dramatic results by switching back and forth from close-up to wide-angle, from side view to full-face shots.

> Such an arrangement is what I hypothesize in principle for the brain: multiple circuits (some healthy, some pathogenic) arranged in sets that operate simultaneously—but with only one circuit (of a set) at a time having access to a particular 'final common pathway' (of neural, neuroendocrine, and neuroimmune mechanisms) that innervates and influences a particular body system, organ, class of tissue or cells, enzymes, and so forth. Although only one circuit at a time can have access to the outflow path connected with its set, the system allows for switching from one to another. (p. 207)

Besides rapid cycling among bipolar patients, Reiser points to the following phenomena which share similar characteristics in terms of the rapidity of their on- and offset: abrupt onset of night terrors, abrupt onset and cessation of epileptic seizures, rapid and dramatic changes in the states of consciousness associated with the induction and termination of hypnotic states, abrupt and sudden onset of episodes of narcolepsy and cataplexy, disappearance of striatal rhythmic tremors and rigidity of Parkinsonism and choreoathetotic movements of tardive dyskinesia during sleep and their reappearance with awakening, sudden death following taboo violations among primitive people, rapid onset of psychotic behaviors in mass group phenomena such as lynching, sudden abrupt changes of personality in patients with multiple personalities, sudden abrupt onset and cessation of fugues and hysterical dissociative states, etc. Such sudden switches in the usage of circuits are not only pathological formations, they are also part of healthy living, as for example in the case of normal REM cycles and other biorhythms.

Thus, it may be said that a person who slips into psychosis does not really invent a whole new person, or a whole new way of being, feeling, and thinking. Rather, preexisting different parts of the self, parts that normally lie dormant or are unconscious, are activated. Multiple personalities, though not psychotic, are a particularly striking example. One personality, Tim, drinks orange juice with no ill effect, while Tom has an allergic reaction such as hives. As long as the juice is still digested the hives are present; however, as soon as Tim returns, they disappear. In a multiple personality the different persona have different personalities, memories, handwritings, talents, knowledge of foreign languages and right- or left-handedness. Depending on which personality operates, rashes, scars, and other tissue injuries will be present or absent, responses to drugs and their dosage may vary, and visual acuity and blood pressure readings may vary significantly. Something like it, though not as extreme, can happen in affective disorders: The circuits involved in a depressed mood, in cognition, or in remembering, are available to all of us; but it takes specific provocations to activate them and to make them the predominant circuits. People who are diagnosed as depressives can be thought of, among other things, as having defective or ineffective mechanisms with which to mediate stress. In order to make sense out of this proposition we have to return to the question of how affect regulations are acquired—or how the organism can fail to acquire them.

Jay Weiss's (1972) experiment with induced helplessness in rats will serve as an illustration of the mechanisms leading to such an hypothesis. He took two sets of rats and put them into adjacent cages. Both sets of animals were subjected to identical electric shocks, and for the same length of time. However, one group of rats could see a light go on just before the shock would happen, thereby giving these rats a chance to do something to change their fate, namely by learning to turn off the shock as soon as they saw the light (operant conditioning—active avoidance). Since both cages received the shocks simultaneously and from the same source, the first group in effect determined the amount and duration of the second shock not only for themselves but the second group as well. However, there was one major difference: While the externally induced stress—the shock—was identical for both groups, the first group, A, learned that their actions, i.e., their ability to learn, could be highly effective, while the second group, B, merely learned behavioral despair, one of the basic cognitive-affective sets that underlies depression. As a consequence, group B developed significantly more stomach ulceration, lost more weight, had higher levels of the stress hormone corticosterone in its bloodstream, and became more fearful. In other words, the rats in group B had become perfect candidates for major depressive episodes and for psychosomatic diseases. Conversely, in group A, which escaped fairly unscathed, the experience of having been in control of their fate established a complex psychophysiological set of responses that acted as a protective mechanism capable of mediating the most severe effects of their shocking adventure, at least on their stomach walls.

If these relationships did not also occur in the wild, Weiss's experiments might be fairly meaningless. And even though, in the wild, conditions are not very hard to find they are extremely difficult to quantify. However, Sapolsky (1987) succeeded; he found the analog among olive baboons in the wild-life preserve of the Serengeti. We have known for some time that among humans as well as apes, executives, i.e., those who can exercise some control over their fates, are better equipped to deal with stress than are their subordinates. What Sapolsky found was a particular troop where six of the highest-ranking males had succeeded in eliminating the leader of the troop. In the months that followed, the question of succession was never settled; instead there was a pronounced degree of social instability, where ranks shifted daily. Aggression rose, sexual encounters declined, and alliances were formed and abandoned in rapid succession. In short, all the usual psychological advantages of dominance, such as having a predictable and stable position in society, vanished. The top males still dominated the troop and they were well-fed and in the prime of life. But instead of enjoying the healthy physiology of the dominant males they had been and of the one they had displaced, they showed elevated hydrocortisone levels, their stress responses were sluggish and poorly regulated, and they had difficulty maintaining testosterone levels during periods of stress. These findings are critical. Besides confirming or supporting the findings of Weiss's experiments, they show that in the *wilds* a behavioral state— holding a position of dominance—can affect physiology, i.e., the ability to mediate stress, depending on the circumstances in which the stress occurs. It seems that the way in which dominance affects health depends on the degree to which the world is experienced as being secure and predictable for the individuals at the top of a hierarchy.

These findings also provide an excellent paradigm for both Reiser's concept of affective illness and the major psychoses as "stress disorders," and for psychotherapy as the attempt to teach an old brain new tricks. But how?

Now we have to go back even further: Anxiety as a signal is an inborn mechanism in man and beast alike. So is the ability to anticipate danger and the capacity to mobilize defensive maneuvers to alleviate the painful experience and to defend against it. Indeed, Kandel has argued that the cortical development that facilitates the ability to imagine and to defend against all possible dangers that may lie ahead had an evolutionary advantage. Tiger advanced the same argument for the ability to hope. Simplified, we may say: "She who saw the Ice Age coming, and who looked for a nice warm cave, had the largest number of surviving grandchildren." In the course of evolution, homo sapiens also developed the capacity to react to dangers emanating from inside himself and to defend against them with the mental and physiological equivalent of fight or flight. "He who kicked a tree trunk, instead of his mother, was rewarded with the woman who found the warm cave."

In our chapter dealing with the etiology of affective disorders we discussed the concept of "object constancy," the infant's ability to retain a sense of mother's presence even in her absence. Now we can easily imagine two psychophysiological scenarios: one, where the receding steps of the caretaker produce signal anxiety, then protest, then a grasping for the transitional object and, as a consequence, a shift into a memory pathway that conjures up sensations of being soothed and calmed. In the second scenario, the same sounds of receding steps results in a sequence that leads from signal anxiety to protest to behavioral despair, with no available memory traces of soothing and with no psychophysiological means to mediate the stress experience. While, admittedly, this is an exceedingly crude or simplified model of the biology of object constancy, it may offer a useful grasp of the phenomenon. For something very much like it takes place.

The structure of the neural network capable of receiving, evaluating, coding, storing, and retrieving this kind of informational input notably involves the locus ceruleus (LC), two small nuclei situated bilaterally in the brainstem which are part of the norepinephrine system (NE). These small nuclei provide more than 70% of the total norepinephrine produced in the primate brain and thus indirectly control a large part of the peripheral sympathetic nervous system. While our understanding of the workings of this alarm relay system is by no means complete, we do know that it exists and that it acts as a filter for the sensations of fear and pain. Overactivity of this nucleus is associated with morbid anxiety states (as differentiated from panic disorders), while lesions in this area produce the opposite, namely a dulling of these sensations. The LC-NE system has an exquisite two-way communication with the association cortex and the limbic system, in other words, with the systems that evaluate the meaning of incoming stimuli and their associational connections with the memories of past events.

According to both Reiser and Willner, responses to psychological and physiological stresses can be thought of as occurring in four stages: (1) recognition and evaluation of danger; (2) transduction; (3) activation of CNS stress mechanisms; and (4) pathophysiological sequelae in organs and tissues. What we call signal anxiety, then, occurs between stages 1 and 3 and probably overlaps with parts of each. The LC-NE system is genetically shaped, but is influenced by experience and learning. As small children we want to play in traffic until we learn better. Therapy, any therapy which aims at real changes in the way we react to stress, would have to be able to teach the organism to learn from experience in the same way that Weiss's rats learned by controlling electric shocks. The day will come when a call from mother-in-law only causes mild concern. Yet how do we get there and how does what we have learned in the last several decades about the workings of the brain help to accomplish this goal?

First of all, we have to point out emphatically what our new understanding cannot lead to: Obviously, none of what has been reported so far is meant to suggest that there is a brave new world of psychotherapy right around the corner where we can simply forge optimistic new pathways into patients' heads via electrical stimulation or other utopian methods. To the contrary, by having working models of how mental or behavioral habits are reflections of neuronal activity and vice versa, we are becoming more appreciative of the necessity of time and repetition in the therapeutic endeavor. When we say now that a "maladaptive pattern" is "deeply ingrained," we have a much better understanding of what that means, and we have a better idea of why this presents a real problem as opposed to a "mere failure of nerve" on the part of the patient. This knowledge contradicts many of the traditional and contemporary bootstrap theories of psychotherapy, even pedagogy. "Getting it" is not stress-induced divine revelation. It is unlikely to come bursting through in a single loud primal scream. If useful revelation occurs, it is most likely to represent the end point of a long process of cognitive, motivational, and behavioral reeducation.

Generally, all three systems just mentioned "hang together." A chronically enraged, suspicious, depressed patient typically has thought processes and belief systems to match his behavioral repertoire and vice versa. And it is with those "sets" that he or she approaches psychotherapy or EST, the family physician, voodoo, or the parish priest. If any of these individuals or institutions appeal to the person with problems, if their sets match, then therapy, whatever its nature may be, psychoanalysis or a "hex," will work. This also holds true if the family physician prescribes a starch compound called Hope-ophetamine, or when the new AA member turns his life over to a Higher Power. Several mechanisms are at work here: to list just the most important ones—placebo effect, catharsis, and simply the relationship between two people, one of whom is adjudicated to be wiser, stronger, and more powerful. The activation of a transference, i.e., the attribution of wished-for qualities onto another human being, operates not only in the analytic situation but in just about any human interaction, particularly when it involves a status differential, be it real or imaginary.

It is precisely at the point when individuals are at their wits' end in terms of feeling competent to help themselves, that he or she seeks out somebody who is more knowledgeable and more powerful. Initially just about any therapist or therapy will help, and it does not matter whether the therapeutic mode involves the talking cure or the relics of a saint. After all, it is worth remembering that with all the advanced scientific knowledge which the West so proudly possesses, non-Western societies are still considerably more effective in containing the major mental illnesses in non-asylum settings than we are. In fact, in some instances it is precisely some form of voodoo or magical intervention that is all that is called for in terms of treatment. For example, a fairly common occurrence among soldiers during World War I was a disorder which was known as "stocking paralysis." Battle-fatigued soldiers would appear in infirmaries with one or two partially paralyzed legs. Typically, the prescription was for sugar pills and the army physician would then take something resembling a Magic Marker, and with it draw on the skin a circular line, one or two inches above the ankle around the soldier's leg (that is why it was called stocking paralysis). The doctor would then instruct the patient to faithfully take his pills in order for sensations and motion to return in his legs within a matter of days, but only up to that magic line that had been drawn: no more and no less. Once that point was reached, another line would be drawn, another few inches up, and in this fashion normal sensations and movements returned inch by inch, line by line. Obviously, any conventional medical justification for this approach is a physiological impossibility, given the fact that one muscle which extends from the ankle to the knee cannot possibly be paralyzed in that fashion. But since the average army recruit during that time typically did not possess this kind of anatomical knowledge, the treatment of being listened to, the doctor's validation of the complaint, sympathetic noises from all around, and the institution of a few days of R & R worked very well indeed. It simply was not necessary in most of those cases to address the real cause of the paralysis—namely, battle fatigue. In this day and age, weary employees simply decide to take what they call a "mental health day." It seems that magical skin markings, a day at the races, or an afternoon at Elizabeth Arden's, should they accomplish the desired cure, probably work via the same neuronal pathways.

The majority of patients suffering from clinical depression, however, suffer from more than just battle fatigue or shell shock, though they may suffer from that too. Besides childhood trauma, they bring to the situation layers of defensive modes and structures, a compulsion to replay the original family drama, selective cognitive filters, and last but not least, real life experiences. Taken together, these form the complex formation of the adult psyche with all its strengths and weaknesses. It is also an unfortunate fact of life that many of the most ingenious survival techniques that allow children to grow in some fashion even in the most gruesome environments, turn out to be quite maladaptive—even counterproductive—in adult life. Put differently, it is one of the central paradoxes of human psychology that the ingenuity of the survivor may also pose the most difficult therapeutic problem.

The victim, once he is an adult, often becomes his own worst enemy. For example, Samuel Pisar (1979), internationally renowned legal scholar and peace activist, had had an extremely traumatic childhood. When he was ten, he lived for two years under an oppressive antisemitic Russian occupation. During that time his father disappeared. When the Germans replaced the Russians, occupying this part of Poland, they began to round up Jews systematically. His mother and sister were sent to Auschwitz where they were gassed immediately. Samuel also ended up in Auschwitz, and then in four additional concentration camps in the course of the next four years (ages 12–16). Sheer physical survival became the challenge of his adolescence. What protected him and helped him to survive—besides a great deal of luck—were two things. First was the magical belief that his mother had known intuitively how to save his life. On the day of the transport she had chosen to dress him in long pants rather than short ones; consequently, he was classified as an adult instead of a child, which meant that instead of being gassed, he was put to work. Second, he attached himself to two other adolescents, slightly older than himself, and together they formed a little posse or gang—a protective family. According to his autobiography, this experience also taught him how to be shrewd, cunning, ruthless, and deceitful. Following liberation, the very skills which had enabled these youngsters to survive Auschwitz had also prepared them for careers as successful black marketeers. Thus, they found themselves in an American army prison within a year of having been liberated by this very army. Eventually, it was a prolonged physical illness which gave Pisar the opportunity to drastically rethink his entire life and to grow up all over again. This time around, however, he grew into the ethical man we now admire.

Pisar's story is in stark contrast to that of Burt: Burt grew up with an alcoholic and extremely abusive father. When he was old enough to fight back, his father arranged it so that he was made a warden of the state and he spent the next five years (ages 13–18) in several of New York City's finest mental institutions. Since these hospitals agreed with the family, that it was the boy who was the one with the problem, it was decided to "rehabilitate" him. As a result, Burt became the all-time expert in fighting off all intrusions, be they psychotherapy, psychotropic drugs, or educational efforts. Unfortunately, this very expertise became the major obstacle to his psychotherapy as an adult, once he himself decided he needed it. It manifested itself in what can only be described as hypervigilance, a need to prove over and over again that he was immune to outside influences. What finally mobilized him to utilize the therapeutic situation in a more productive way was his therapist's suggestion that he should stop treatment until such time as he was ready to really work on himself.

Since affective disorders are never a single entity but a syndrome consisting of cognition, affect, and interpersonal dynamics, psychotherapy has to address all three of these dimensions in order to be effective. On the most basic level, a good part of the depressed population is simply lonely. This may be due to circumstances such as old age and a move to an unfamiliar place, lack of social skills or, alternatively, deep-rooted intrapsychic conflicts or a mixture of all three. As mentioned earlier, research has shown that, on the average, what is called "social skills training," for female outpatients suffering from moderate degrees of unipolar depression, is slightly more effective than antidepressant medication. Obviously, depression and social isolation mutually reinforce each other. What these studies indicate, then, is that the lack of social skills in making friends, in maintaining social support systems, and the resulting loneliness, are as least as important in causing depression as biological causes or deep-rooted intrapsychic conflicts.

Burt, for example, who had been robbed of normal adolescence and consequently of the social skills and the friends that are normally acquired during that time period, grew into adult-

hood with the social graces of a cave man. That does not mean
that in his case a Dale Carnegie course could have been an
adequate substitute for psychotherapy; still, it would have been
a valuable adjunct to the psychotherapy and the antidepressant
medication which he did in fact need. Having severed all contact
with his family, and furthermore, having acquired no friends
(though he kept in touch with some of his former fellow-in-
mates), Burt led a very isolated and lonely life. Alcohol and
drugs became the substitutes for social and emotional connections.

Given the incidence of divorce in our society, and given the
fact that, on the average, American adults make 14 geographic
moves in the course of their adult lives, the problem of loneliness is not one to dismiss easily. Being lonely has to be distinguished from being alone. A person can be just as lonely in a
group of people as when alone. Loneliness is a state of feeling
unconnected to other people, of wanting to be with someone
who is not there, of having no one to turn to who can affirm our
essential human qualities. Then there is the emotional loneliness earmarked by the absence of an intimate attachment, such
as a love relationship, a "best friend," or a marriage, and then
there is the social loneliness which is characterized by the absence of a community or network of friends to whom one feels
attached. Though everybody can feel intensely lonely at some
point in his or her lives, there are also people who are chronically lonely and they differ in some quite important ways from
those who are not, or who only encounter the problem occasionally. Typically, the chronically lonely blame themselves, their
lack of attractiveness or intelligence for their isolation and—
equally important—they do not like most people they meet who
could be potential friends. The question whether those people
would find *them* attractive, is then really academic, after all "who
would want to belong to a club that would have me as a member" is not a question that can be answered readily.

Chronically lonely people also often lack simple social skills,
such as how to introduce themselves, how to communicate, and

how to issue a simple invitation for tea. They also tend to talk about themselves more than others, ask fewer questions about the person they are talking to, and in the course of any conversation they switch topics more often then their more gregarious and outgoing counterparts. The chronically lonely are either too reluctant to discuss subjects that may prove to be self-revealing or, alternatively, they reveal too much, too soon, and too fast with the result that their targets back away from what they experience as an avalanche of intimate information. Unfortunately it can often be the very pain of prolonged loneliness that causes them to be so self-involved, so greedy for being seen or heard, which makes them such undesirable conversational partners. The anguish associated with feelings of not really mattering to anybody accentuates the narcissism, thus setting a vicious cycle in motion. Additionally, since the needs of such people are usually bottomless, given their history of self-isolation, they have now entirely unrealistic expectations about what friendships can do, hopes that cannot possibly be met, thereby setting the stage for repeated disappointments. Small offenses on the part of potential friends are experienced as abusive interactions or expressions of contempt. Consequently, chronically lonely people back out faster from evolving relationships than do others. Any person or interaction that does not live up to their exaggerated standards of what love relationships and friendships should be like is therefore readily dismissed as unworthy. Then again, they frantically search for the idealized relationship and in the course of this search they neglect the pursuit of multiple friendships that would not be so taxing.

In a therapy setting these problems can be quite difficult to address. Group therapy is ideally suited for that purpose; it allows for the gentle and slow identification of behavior patterns that tend to alienate other people. It also offers immediate rewards for the learning of more attractive ways of interacting and communicating. But if, for whatever reason, a chronically lonely and depressed person cannot or will not become a member of a group, and if that person is entirely unaware of his or her contribution to their isolation, how is the therapeutic interaction to address this painful subject? This is particularly poignant when self-involvement and self-consciousness are already the principal problems. In those cases it can be quite a delicate matter to bring this to someone's attention without making them feel even more self-conscious or ashamed than they already are. In addition, very often the only data that the therapist has available are those generated by the therapeutic interaction, the transference. This poses a considerable problem because, justifiably, the point can be made that these data, i.e., the nature of the interaction, should *not* be used to make such a point, because the therapeutic setting is *the one* situation where an individual is supposed to make the self the main focus of inquiry.

Burt sometimes spun out fantasies, and once joked about a cottage industry designed to freeze-dry dead pets. This he did on the day when, for the first time in her life, Eurydice, the office terrier, lay on the floor, running a fever and obviously ill. Burt is probably one of the most generous people I have ever met. In a blizzard, he would not have a moment's hesitation to personally carry the sick pooch of a friend clear across town if that was where the only vet was to be found. Against this characterological backdrop, his remarks and the timing of them, had to be addressed. The therapist, who was also the incensed owner of the dog, readily agreed with Burt that the therapy session was supposed to be *only about* the patient, not the injured feelings of the therapist. He certainly had the *right* to express whatever feelings he might have, without fear of censure. In Burt's eyes, censure would have been a breach of therapeutic contract. On the other hand, he had to understand that such deliberate expressions of sadism also constitute, among other things, a message about how that patient feels about intimacy and closeness and about its attendant dangers. He needed to know that the point of my communication to him was not to judge the morality of his position but to point out what its effects might be on another person. Besides, it has to be a desperately lonely place that would prompt associations such as his. Grudgingly,

Burt conceded the point, allowing us then to address his conflicts pertaining to loneliness.

Studies which have compared the effectiveness of different schools of psychotherapy and their corresponding techniques for the treatment of depression have identified two approaches as being most successful: cognitive therapy and interpersonal psychotherapy. These two approaches represent two distinct and separate schools of thought; however, it seems to make more sense not to compare these two schools (or their content and modus operandi) of doing psychotherapy, but to simply discuss the way therapy (by any name) can evaluate and address the cognitive, intrapsychic, and interpersonal dimensions of depression.

Clearly, there are differences between the way normal people process information and the way depressed people do. To wit: Once upon a time there were two frogs. Both of them fell into a pail of milk. Frog A said, "I knew this would happen—no sense in fighting fate." Frog B said, "I have a co-op in Florida and I will not let this little misfortune keep me from retiring there." And with that thought, Frog B began to paddle furiously. Twelve hours later, Frog A was dead, while Frog B sat on a lump of butter. The moral of that story is obvious, since it captures a great deal of the essence of the depressive mode of thinking.

Yapko (1988) has identified the following dimensions of depressed cognitive functioning: negative expectations (hopelessness), negative self-evaluation, negative interpretation of events, suicidal ideation, indecision, confusion, primarily internal focus, diminished concentration span, primarily past temporal orientation, global thinking style, "victim mind set" (helplessness), cognitive distortions (erroneous patterns of thinking), rumination, perceptual amplification, and rigidity (p. 29). Furthermore, as Aaron Beck (1967) has shown, these cognitive patterns are usually automatic and involuntary.

For example, how did Frog A "know" that he would wind up in a pail of milk, that the fates had decided that he would end his days in such an undignified fashion, unless he had had that very same thought every time something went wrong? Would this frog look upon the lump of butter as a lifesaver or as a threat to his cholesterol level? Probably the latter. This pessimistic frog's autobiography, then, is scripted in such a way as to confirm over and over again that the world is (for him) unsafe, that nothing good will ever happen to him, and all new events and images must be interpreted as confirmations of his basic premise. Such cognitive sets, painful and unrewarding as they may seem, are not all bad for the person who uses them. They do have their advantages or, as we like to say, they have "secondary gains." First of all, they make life quite predictable, since the outcome of all efforts is guaranteed from the outset. Risks are all but eliminated. Secondly, by construing a life this way, the author of it is in full control. Instead of being judged, he does the judging; instead of being the victim, he becomes the savvy agent of his own fate. Here nothing is left to chance. If I have already told the whole world just how stupid I am, I cannot possibly make a fool out of myself. In other words, in dealing with the cognitive sets of a patient we are not dealing with something akin to a simple misunderstanding, but with a safety net that to him is often experienced as being vital. It may well be the only way in which the patient knows how to survive and to be in this world safely.

Such positions are not surrendered easily. In fact, they are often fiercely defended as the only appropriate way to deal with reality. To take the risk of trying on a new, and therefore potentially dangerous reality, requires a bit of trust; this, in turn, can only evolve on the basis of a sound "working alliance" between the therapist and the patient. These two people have to have a history together in which the therapist has acted reliably and repeatedly in the patient's best interests. Before addressing the more complex aspects of this interaction, it bears repeating: What cures in the therapeutic enterprise is the *relationship* between the two people rather than what either one of them *does*.

Obviously, then, that relationship has to be stable, dependable, ongoing, and it has to be defined by parameters that are based on an almost contractual arrangement. The predictability and the continuity of this venture are vital. To meet once a week, or preferably twice, is absolutely essential if any real work is to be accomplished. This recommendation should become more plausible if we go back to the problem of object constancy.

People who as small infants did not have a reliable enough "object" or human "other" cannot acquire it in adulthood through insight alone. Unless they are induced to form an attachment and to allow themselves to depend on at least some aspect of the therapeutic relationship if not the therapist him- or herself, they cannot build the missing structures that allow them to properly deal with separation. For this to take place, the very experience of meeting every Tuesday and Friday at three o'clock (but not on other days), week in and week out, is something that lends itself as tangibly as a block to building an enduring image and the expectation that the "object" will continue to exist even in its absence. Infants and patients cannot risk attaching themselves to a phantom, a fleeting presence, or to an oppressive, ever-present object. There has to be a balance between the extremes of deprivation and suffocating excess; quantity does not serve for quality (in primal interactions especially), nor can quality make up for infrequency or undependability.

The psychoanalytic term "evenly hovering attention" denotes fairly accurately the midpoint between detachment and symbiosis. Most important, however, is the fact that the interaction has parameters that are predictable. For example, therapy hours can only be changed by mutual consent. In another book (Schad-Somers, 1982) I have referred to the process by which patients learn to rely on the predictable presence of the therapist as "taming." This term has been borrowed from de Saint-Exupéry's moving fable *The Little Prince*. In his travels through the different planets, the Little Prince finally lands on earth. In his search for a friend he eventually encounters a fox. Having only lived a solitary existence and not knowing anything about relationships, the Little Prince asks for instant friendship. Thus the fox has to explain to him that in order to be friends, the Little

Prince has to tame him first. The ensuing dialogue deserves quoting in full, since nothing I know captures the initial encounter between total strangers more poetically than de Saint-Exupéry has done:

"No," said the Little Prince. "I am looking for friends. What does that mean, 'tame'?"

"It is an act too often neglected," said the fox. "It means to establish ties."

"'To establish ties'?"

"Just that," said the fox. "To me you are still nothing more than a little boy who is just like a hundred thousand other little boys. And I have no need of you. And you, on your part, have no need of me. To you I am nothing more than a fox like a hundred thousand other foxes. But if you tame me, then we shall need each other. To me you will be unique in all the world. To you, I shall be unique in all the world. . ."

"I am beginning to understand," said the Little Prince. "There is a flower . . . I think that she has tamed me. . ."

"It is possible," said the fox. . . "My life is very monotonous," he said. "I hunt chickens; men hunt me. All the chickens are just alike, and all the men are just alike. And, in consequence, I am a little bored. But if you tame me, it will be as if the sun came to shine on my life. I shall know the sound of a step that will be different from all others. Other steps send me hurrying back underneath the ground. Yours will call me, like music, out of my burrow. And then, look: you see the grain fields down yonder? I do not eat bread. Wheat is of no use to me. And that is sad. But you have hair that is the color of gold. Think how wonderful that will be when you have tamed me! The grain, which is also golden, will bring me back to the thought of you. And I shall love to listen to the wind in the wheat. . ."

The fox gazed at the little prince, for a long time.

"Please—tame me!" he said.

"I want to very much," the Little Prince replied. "But I have not much time. I have friends to discover, and a great many things to understand."

"One only understands the things one tames," said the fox. "Men have no more time to understand anything. They buy things already made at the shops. But there is no shop anywhere where one can buy friendship, and so men have no friends anymore. If you want a friend, tame me. . ."

"What must I do to tame you?" asked the Little Prince.

"You must be very patient," replied the fox. "First you will sit down at a little distance from me—like that—in the grass. I shall look at you out of the corner of my eye, and you will say nothing. Words are the source of misunderstandings. But you will sit a little closer to me, every day. . ."

The next day the Little Prince came back.

"It would have been better to come back at the same hour," said the fox. "If, for example, you come at four o'clock in the afternoon, then at three o'clock I shall begin to be happy. I shall feel happier and happier as the hour advances. At four o'clock, I shall already be worrying and jumping about. I shall show you how happy I am! But if you come at just any time, I shall never know at what hour my heart is to be ready to greet you. . . . One must observe the proper rites. . ." (pp. 66–68)

For the color of wheat to serve sufficiently as the symbolic representation of the other is what, in the therapeutic enterprise, we strive for in the process of establishing "object constancy." Typically, during the initial stages of therapy, depressed patients have no visual, acoustic, or tactile memory of either the therapist, the office, or the chair they sat on. For some, the therapist ceases to exist altogether between sessions or during the therapist's vacation. The fact that Samuel Pisar was able to retain a visible image of his mother, not the one he saw leaving with his sister for the ovens, but the one who wisely chose long pants for him, and that, therefore, he could think of as guarding him, clearly indicates that the mother-son attachment here had been secure and loving, one capable of protecting the child from depression, and in this case, literally death by demoralization.

What makes the process of establishing object constancy in adulthood different from a simple learning process is the fact that in the case of a grown person we are not dealing affectively and cognitively with a clean slate. The patient for whom we cease to exist cannot be thought of as merely missing a tape, or a message on the tape, or as being passive. To the contrary, something else took the place of object constancy, something that can lead quite an active life. The patient who feels that I am dead between sessions has metaphorically to kill me off and then resurrect me twice a week. Even more complex, the patient who drove six hours to get to New York on Thanksgiving Day, only to find her therapist's office closed, was setting up an elaborate scenario. Before the patient, who actually did this, became thoroughly depressed, she said to herself, "I knew this would happen," at the same time being entirely unaware that her "knowing" was a consequence of her own arranging it that way. However, her cognitive set of "victim," though necessary to her, is not sufficient in this instance to explain that a certain "something" (in the form of an attitude both manipulative and self-destructive) had developed in the absence of a secure attachment.

Given what we have already noted about the etiology of mood disorders, it is impossible to summarize their intrapsychic and interpersonal aspects and do justice to the complexity of the subject. After all, there are as many reasons why people become depressed as there are depressed persons, and no two are alike. However, in terms of intrapsychic causality, two interrelated clusters stand out: (1) insufficient, ambivalent, or malignant attachments; and (2) narcissistic disturbances. These two clusters are related in a way that is similar to the relationship between the dollar and the yen: they are both determined by a common world economy, and they are the products of two separate national economies.

One particular therapy session should illustrate the point. Mary is exquisitely sensitive to criticism, and she is equally vulnerable to abandonments, particularly on the part of her therapist, who functions as her self object, her lifeline. In order to feel real, and good about herself, Mary needs an affirming other. The therapy session I am about to describe took place on a Tuesday following Memorial Day. The loneliness generated by a long weekend had turned Mary into a telephone answering machine abuser, who called so often that the message tape ran out, leaving no room for further messages. She had felt abandoned, furious, and she retaliated by initiating a malignant interaction. With the Bell Telephone slogan, "Let your fingers do the walking" she had almost complete power over one important aspect of my life. Needless to say, I must rely on my phone a great deal, and since she knew I was out of town, doing something about the effectiveness of my machine obviously presented a considerable difficulty for me. Pretty heady stuff, indeed. The excitement generated by the commission of this "crime" acted at least temporarily as a powerful "antidepressant." For the time it took Mary to screw up the electronic works, she reveled in her power to counteract my rotten act of leaving her with her ability to cut me off from all other patients. Mary's index finger had turned into a dangerous weapon.

The following session (or one out of four possible scripts, given the same circumstances) begins with Mary putting on her most endearing, disarming smile, and announcing, in the sincerest of voices, "I really want to apologize for the phone calls, but don't want to discuss this right now—I have important stuff to talk about and I want to buckle down immediately and make this a good working session." Thirty-second pause. Then, "You should be very proud of me, because for the first time since I have been in therapy I did not. . . ." (fill in the blank with familiar varieties of acting out). What Mary is asking for, if not demanding, is praise for refraining from a fictional deed that she could have committed, but chose not to. In other words, I have just been handed the job of repairing her damaged self-esteem, to make her feel good about herself, to erase the shame over the phone calls. Now, I know from experience that as long as my eyes remain focused on her and as long as they do not communicate my anger, we will continue—at least for a while—to interact in a nonpsychotic fashion. I have to choose between keeping my eyes focused and taking a walk in my head. If my eyes drift, Mary will shift into the psychotic mode, choosing between four possible tracks: (1) "I am dropping out of therapy . . ."; (2) "My lawyer will sue you for . . . . You can expect papers to be served by . . . ."; (3) "I think you should take responsibility for the fact that your therapy group is disintegrating—I have done some research, and I know it is entirely unethical for a therapist to allow patients to meet outside of group," and (4) "I finally realize that your relationship with your patients is ruled only by one thing: by how much money you need for your fancy beach house." All four of these programs, or "tapes," have a minimum duration of 35 minutes, which means that in the course of a 45-minute session I shall have five minutes to rescue her, two minutes for her to apologize, and another three minutes for me to console and praise her enough for her to be able to leave the session with her head held high. If I were to refuse to play my part, the tapes could run for weeks on end and they would eventually converge into one final common pathway, which is: "I am terminating therapy and I am moving in with my mother."

How, in this admittedly extreme, though not at all exaggerated example, can the talking cure accomplish anything? Needless to say, without proper medication, talking will achieve absolutely nothing useful. But, assuming Mary is pharmacologically stabilized, there are two developmental tasks that therapy has to address. In terms of her way of relating to others, she has to learn and really come to believe that no one human being can meet all her dependency needs, that there are other people in the world, and that she can find ways to alleviate her loneliness that do not involve either her therapist or her mother or her work. Secondly, Mary has to learn that I cannot be in charge of the job of regulating her self-esteem, that there are other sources, such as friends, school, volunteer work, and that ultimately Mary herself will have to learn to give herself praise when praise is due.

I have always found that group therapy is invaluable in facilitating developmental tasks of the magnitude that Mary had to accomplish. To make this possible, a group has to be stable, ongoing, long-term, and committed. For Mary, group therapy has primarily three functions. First of all, as she is fiercely competitive, "group" represents a major challenge to her. She wants to be the one who accumulates the largest number of emotional improvement credits. Secondly, since she is also running for the "most insightful co-therapist" award, she has to focus on and pay attention to psyches other than her own. Last, not least, the group functions for her as a safety net, people she can talk to, meet, phone, colleagues who function essentially as a substitute family.

If we take Mary's infamous Tuesday session as the prototype of her emotional problems, we might raise the questions of how one could bring Mary to the point where such an impasse moves ahead, how she might change direction, or how a quite predictable sequence might be shortened. First of all, the malignant telephone connection was an eventuality for which the two of us together were responsible. Originally, phone calls had served the function of seeing Mary through crises and hard times. However, as her breakdown progressed she began to associate the telephone with the experience of mania or madness in general. Even a call that may have originated in a genuine desire to feel better would eventually switch into psychotic mania. It had become a conditioned response, one which kept her crazy, provided excitement, and allowed her to stay in a space where she did not have to deal with the task of facing the consequences of her malignant and destructive behavior patterns. Unfortunately, I had been unaware of this development until after it had been firmly established. Then it became clear that nothing could be accomplished until the telephone connection was severed completely. Consequently, Mary's phone privileges were withdrawn entirely. I told her that if she called, I would simply hang up. What followed was a very slow and painful learning experience. Once the phone connection was gone, it left Mary no choice but to find excitement and stimulation someplace else. Furthermore, what was entirely missing in Mary's behavioral and emotional repertoire was sadness, the ability to cry because the absent object is, at least for the moment, lost. Apparently very early in Mary's infancy this particular way of communicating was extinguished or buried. Mary had to be taught to cry out of sadness, a response that came progressively faster with practice. Tears became the signal for a return to sanity and the renewed contact with the lost object. This took several years. But if we consider that this particular emotional expression, which is so fundamental, had probably gotten lost during the first year of life, that her brain and her mind had developed without having access to these feelings, it should not be too surprising that this process took as long as it did.

But now, after another long weekend, and with another summer approaching, I find a letter from her in the mailbox which says, "I am numb when I think I will not see you for two months. . . . please don't go. . . . On the radio they are playing a beautiful Mozart dance. So simple & graceful & moving." She continues, "You did the right thing by not answering my calls. I have to learn that what we do in my session cannot be combatted the next day by a phone call, like the old times. Sad, sad that I wasted $2/3$ of my session yesterday." Clearly, things are shifting in Mary's head. She knows that Mozart is just about my favorite composer, she owns a record set of Gluck's *Orfeo et Euridice*; in other words, she is finding her own version of the "color of wheat."

With respect to the problem of allowing attachments to take place, or rather to consciously acknowledge that they exist and that they matter, patients such as Burt and Bernie have similar, yet quite different sets of problems. Burt's standard response to my vacation, initially, was "Good riddance, go with God, but go—it saves me a lot of money." Bernie always assured me that I deserved time off, that it gave him more time to get his writing done, and that he was after all a grown man rather than a dependent child. Clearly, Bernie had learned early in life not to let other people come too close or matter too much, while Burt had experienced all caregiving individuals as outright dangerous. Whatever history a patient brings to therapy, it has to be understood, interpreted; an effort has to be made to counter the original traumatic experience with one that is better. The new way of "being with" can then, step by step, be incorporated into the cognitive, affective, and behavioral repertoire of the patient until eventually he or she learns to say:

"No, I had no way of knowing this would happen. But I will find a way to deal with it."

Special Problems
Stigma, Shame, and Suicide

The concept of pharmacological mood regulation is the stuff that dreams and movies are made of. Unfortunately, most of them are either nightmares or horror films. On the other hand, "make it all good again" is the plea on the part of an innocent child who trusts that the parents have such benign and magical powers and that they can exercise them. It is a rare patient who has not, at some point in psychotherapy, uttered the wish that there be some kind of pill to take that would take the place of the painful labor of "working it through." Yet the notion that something malevolent and foreign could take over our brain is probably more frightening a prospect than death. Tales of demonic possession and its exorcism are a standard staple of folklore and fairy tales. Even in our seemingly enlightened age, the movie called *The Exorcist* grossed millions of dollars. Whether it is the devil who takes possession of us or whether it is a hallucinogenic drug that transforms us into Spiderman makes no difference, the experience is the same: something alien has taken over, something that we are unable to control.

For example: "One day this demon was in a high state of delight because he had invented a mirror with this peculiarity: that every good and pretty thing reflected in it shrank away to almost nothing. On the other hand, every bad and good-for-nothing thing stood out and looked its worst. The most beautiful landscapes reflected in it looked like boiled spinach, and the best people became hideous, or else were upside down and had no bodies. Their faces were distorted beyond recognition, and if they had even one freckle it appeared to spread all over the nose and mouth. . . . If a good thought passed through anyone's mind, it turned to a grin in the mirror, and this caused real delight to the demon." This description is remarkably similar to that of Styron's in describing a depressive episode. Alternatively, it could just as well be the description of a "bad trip" on a hallucinogenic mushroom.

It is, however, in Hans Christian Andersen's *The Snow Queen*, where this mirror eventually fell to earth, breaking into billions of fragments, some smaller than grains of sand. If they lodged themselves in the eyes or hearts of people they stuck there and distorted everything they looked at and made them see everything that was amiss. If it got into people's hearts, that heart became like a lump of ice. The victim, a boy by the name of Kay, is helpless; he does not even know that something is wrong. He only knows that the world is ugly and that he no longer loves his little friend Gerda, who follows him to the ends of the earth, to the land of the Snow Queen, to remove that particle from his eye and the one in his heart. Had it not been for her love, Kay would have been condemned to a life of everlasting sorrow. Images such as this are so timeless and enduring because they mirror some of the most profound and universal dreams and terrors. The concept of the magical cure *must* have as its dark underside the threat of demonic transformation. Without the belief in magic, however, the helplessness of childhood could not be endured. Prior to the age of two, an infant has no concept of time. Consequently it experiences pain as pain forever. Without the dimension of time, there exists only "now" and now equals eternity. The crucial difference between the existence in purgatory and in hell is not the severity of the punishment—they are the same—but the element of time. Purgatory is time-limited, hell is not. To be condemned to suffer pain for eternity spells madness. We cannot imagine it. All of us as children experienced this dread, and all of us also remember that some other being or some potion, magically, made it all better. The fascination with and the horror of its power constitute that cluster of attitudes and feelings that propel us forever to follow tyrants, visit Lourdes, buy slimming pills, and fall in love with movie stars. We trade the horror of possession for the dream of salvation.

In Chapter Four I tried to convey how we acquire our reality, just how fragile it really is, and how easily it can become subject to confusion or dissolution; in other words, how easy it is to lose our minds, to go crazy. It is also inherent in the concept of madness that the victim typically does not know it at the time it happens. "Here I was just minding my own business, and the next thing I knew I was locked up in Bellevue Hospital," is a common complaint of people who were hospitalized involuntarily. Sometimes people know it when they are losing touch with reality; typically, they do not. They may simply feel that they are seeing things clearly for the first time. By definition, the ingestion of any *mind-altering* drug, no matter how "minor" it is adjudicated to be, potentially spells craziness. It conjures up pictures of having one's mind manipulated, possibly even in such a way that it will never be the same again. At the same time, it must be remembered that the pain of a depression can be such that the patient would gladly give his eye tooth for some relief. Initially, then, it matters little that a prescription for any psychoactive drug also represents in some ways a disenfranchisement, a surrender of one's autonomy and sovereignty. We adjudicate ourselves as not being fully competent.

A person who previously has been treated with only the talking cure and who then is presented with the recommendation to add medication to the therapeutic regimen, first has to resolve a number of difficult questions pertaining to the "meaning" of that pharmacological intervention with respect to the patient's identity and self-respect. The first question is whether the label "affective disorder" and a prescription for an anti-depressant implies insanity, and stigmatizes the person as a "mental patient," as someone suffering from "mental illness." Secondly, will the medication alter the mind and the brain temporarily or permanently? What will happen to the integrity of the mind? Thirdly, if psychotherapy is supposed to help in "working it through," how can that happen if the mind is manipulated chemically? And, finally, there is the most painful question: Could this possibly be for life, will I ever get entirely well?

Before a pharmacological approach can even be attempted on more than an emergency basis, patients have to first resolve how that fact may alter their identity, self-concept, and their standing as competent adults in their community. The term stigma in this context is used in two ways: one, as an attitude towards the self: "I am a depressive, therefore I am crazy, and I cannot trust myself with anything;" and, two, as a projected attitude towards the self: "People know that I am depressive, therefore nobody will trust me to be responsible."

Furthermore, the introduction of pharmacological agents alters dramatically, at least for the duration of the drug treatment, the relationship between therapist and patient in the direction of even greater inequality. It can do that in two ways. One, it gives the therapist a seemingly irrefutable tool with which to invalidate the patient and, two, it gives the patient a convenient route of escape if the patient chooses to abdicate responsibility and hand the management of the illness over to the therapist. Each of those two possibilities will be addressed in turn.

The problem of stigmatization is particularly difficult in the case of bipolar depression because the entity "manic-depressive insanity," as Bleuler called it, is generally regarded as one of the potentially most severe and essentially incurable forms of mental disturbance. It evokes pictures of the *Son of Sam*, ax-murderers, screeching bag ladies in Grand Central Station, and other terrible pictures of people who are entirely out of control. What the term definitely does *not* conjure up is a rational individual whose judgments can be taken seriously and who can trust his or her own feelings. Perceptions can now be invalidated, patients can be called "crazy," unfit for complex tasks. American voters decided in the case of Senator Eagleton that even two unipolar depressive episodes permanently disqualify an individual from running for the vice presidency. What makes it so difficult to answer the question "what does that mean" is the fact that there are no clear-cut answers. Predictions concerning prognosis of mood-disorders are notoriously unreliable. A best-case scenario would be the following: A depressed patient is given an antidepressant medication, feels better and more resilient to stress, including the stress generated by therapeutic work, which can now progress more rapidly. Everything in the patient's life improves until neither medication nor psychotherapy are needed any more. All ends well. Quite often that does in fact happen. Also, if the bipolar involvement is minor it can easily be controlled by drugs. But there is no guarantee that the biological component will always remain minor, nor does it necessarily mean that it will be present for life. Does a major episode of mania, for example, mean that the individual should not attempt to pursue a very stressful and emotionally demanding career, such as being a psychotherapist or running for public office? The answer is, we don't know. We can state probabilities, such as that 80% of people with such a diagnosis and such treatment had no relapse. But that does not mean that even with the best of treatment, an individual might not fall into the 20% that have relapses or even get worse.

A common approach taken by psychopharmacologists as well as other therapists involved in treating mood disorders is to compare the affective disorder with another chronic physical disorder, such as diabetes, which is also incurable and must be controlled with drugs for the rest of the patient's life. The comparison is meant to make the patient feel better about both the diagnosis and the drug regimen. Unfortunately, presenting the problem in this way also represents a fairly gross mystification of what actually is the case. To call an affective disorder a medical condition like any other disregards the fact that the former involves the patient's sanity, the ability to make rational choices, which may or may not be impaired. The patient knows that very well, and to be told otherwise can be an insult to the person's intelligence.

In order to illustrate just how subtle, complex, and crucial these distinctions can be, the case of Fred provides an excellent example. In the course of many years of treatment this former a-motivational-syndrome, college drop-out with a borderline mode of functioning, had evolved into a very high-functioning individual who had returned to college, gone to graduate school, and become a psychotherapist in private practice. The term "resistance" in Fred's treatment, up until that point, had always only meant one out of two possible things: either Fred was unwilling or unable to face and resolve a particular neurotic conflict or, alternatively, that Fred and his therapist disagreed— again—about something such as values, ethics, politics, etc.— in other words, ordinary, straightforward therapeutic problems that always got resolved.

Then things changed drastically. Fred, who was now in his late 30s, with a life that had become quite stable, became alarmed by the fact that in spite of all this tranquillity he felt chronically overstimulated. Even the activities he enjoyed most felt somewhat painful. Everything was always just a little bit too much. Nothing felt quite right. A neurometric evaluation, a quantitative EEG, helped confirm a diagnosis of bipolar disorder, atypical mania. He was put on very small amounts of Lithium and Tegretol with the hope that in the course of a year or two these drugs could be discontinued. But, for a number of complicated reasons, this is not what happened. His problems got worse, requiring more rather than less medication. During one particularly bad spell, Fred was also given a prescription for small amounts of Navane, an antipsychotic agent, something that Fred clearly recognized he needed. He was aware of the fact that in small ways he had slipped into a mild but nevertheless psychotic state. His thoughts were mildly disordered, so mildly that it would have been unnoticeable to most people. Given Fred's profession, however, he could not afford even the mildest form of thought disorder. The mere fact that Fred the patient, his psychopharmacologist, and his psychotherapist all agreed that at least for a short period of time, he needed a neuroleptic drug, a medication which is designed to control psychosis, has changed his relationship with his therapist subtly, yet in ways that were quite profound and irrevocable.

From now on, Fred has to always at least consider the possibility that at times he may have to rely on his therapists to call his attention to the first signs of his slippage into thought disorder. What that means, among other things, is that now disagreements between Fred and his therapist can be used as potential indicators for his craziness. Matters of opinion now can become much more than that. Suddenly we have a situation where two people who know each other as being extremely opinionated have to work together in such a way that the subjectivity of one in opposition to the subjectivity of another has to also serve as an indicator for thought disorder. The fact that Fred can always use the psychopharmacologist for a second opinion does not really change things for the better. Even if they agree with each other, he still has to trust others that their judgments are accurate. The basic principle, namely that this now constitutes a situation which involves a basic inequality between therapist and patient persists, and cannot be analyzed away.

Usually, a patient who looks back on a psychotic episode which involved hallucinations and delusions, can clearly see the difference between the reality "now" and reality "then." The patient sees it, so does the therapist and the patient's family. But if the slippage into thought disorder is minor, what we see, at least initially, is not lunacy, but merely a patient becoming a bit of a caricature of his or her usual self. For example, in Fred's case, when does a normal passion for clothes become a symptom of mania? One sweater, three sweaters, or a whole new wardrobe? Or simply spending more money than he can afford? How can the patient trust the therapist to "know" when that thin line has been crossed? Who is to know whether we are not simply comparing two sets of prejudices?

While trust is always a sine qua non for all therapeutic work, the quantity and the quality of trust that is required once a mood disorder has progressed to the point where it also involves thought disorder is vastly different. The patient now has to trust two therapists who are using two different data bases, both of which differ from those used by the patient in question. What happens to the judgment of the patient? What if there are contradictory claims with respect to what is "good" for the patient made by family or friends? What are patients to do with what "their gut reaction tells them," or for that matter, their parish priest? Are those judgments to be suspended just because two therapists say so? These questions are impossible to answer. Jack should have trusted his gut reaction because he was in fact given the wrong medication, but he was a "good patient" and up to a point he did as he was told. In another tragic case, a woman with a 20-year history of bipolar disorder and alcoholism improved dramatically with Lithium. But then, under pressure from her local AA chapter, she let her prescription lapse in order not to contradict the anti-drug stance taken by AA. Several months later, on a snowy New Year's night she lay down on the railroad tracks in the village where she had lived all her life.

Not until it was too late did anybody in her family know that for her to survive, medication was absolutely essential. The family also did not know that withdrawal from Lithium—unless it is done very gradually—is a sure prescription for disaster, since sudden withdrawal itself can induce an almost entirely autonomous type of psychosis.

The problem of suicide and its relationship to medication also raises other troubling issues: drug compliance and drug abuse. Sudden withdrawal from many of the drugs discussed here can be a form of passive suicide in that it induces psychosis, and, in the case of amphetamine withdrawal, suicidal depression. In a drug regimen involving Lithium and neuroleptics, even small variations in dosage, or an identical dosage taken at different points in the menstrual cycle, can have a dramatic effect. Almost all patients who are taking psychoactive medications sooner or later will be tempted to experiment a bit. They simply hate the idea of being dependent on "that many drugs," they "forget" to take them, and in the resulting mental confusion they may then in fact forget and take either too many or too few. It is equally common for patients to "forget" to pack the drugs along with other weekend paraphernalia or a business trip together with their papers. Then they may think that a few days won't matter, they may be too ashamed to return from a trip early, lose their prescription, fail to renew an existing one, so their supplies are adequate. Sometimes travelers are separated from their luggage during air travel or they are in a part of the world where their drugs are simply not available. All of these situations can be serious, in fact, life-threatening.

The other side of the coin, namely overdosing, is equally problematic. Many of the central nervous system depressants, as well as most antidepressants, are potentially lethal if a month's supply were to be taken all at once. This would be doubly true if their ingestion is combined with that of alcohol. There is no safe formula for prescriptions, one that is flexible enough to accommodate traveling and accidental loss of medications and one which is safe in that the patient never possesses a potentially lethal dose. Mary, for example, has threatened literally thousands of times to either flush all her medications down the toilet or to take them all at once. The outcome of both actions would probably be identical. Furthermore, the fact that medication relieves the physiological symptoms of mania and depression does not mean that the medicated patient now walks around happy; not at all. Drugs obviously can do nothing in terms of providing people with a life and with the satisfactions that keep other people free from sadness and depression. Social support systems, *confiding, intimate* relationships, have to be acquired first. People who have substituted alcohol or marijuana for a real life, bars for a social life, and dreams for reality will continue to depend on these things even if they are properly medicated.

Closely related to the problem of identity is that of shame. First of all, shame has to be distinguished from guilt. Guilt pertains to doing, shame pertains to being. If I am guilty of a bad deed, I have recourse, I can apologize, I can try to make it up to the other person. A reparative course of action is usually open to me. Shame is a much more archaic reaction than guilt, so primitive that even higher primates and other vertebrae can succumb to it. On one of those lazy August afternoons at the beach, with every human slightly tired and bored, two Coast Guard helicopters evoked four-month-old Eurydice's frenzied fury. Six pounds of puppy fluff noisily chased the helicopters down the entire length of the beach. Just about everybody at that particular stretch of sand burst out laughing at this hilarious spectacle. Everybody then sat up to watch a repeat performance when the helicopters returned. With every eye upon her, Eurydice turned her back to the aircraft and she growled angrily at everybody who tried to goad her into responding to the "big birds." The sight of this pup was both funny and painful, because it so clearly demonstrated the potential pitfalls of infantile grandiosity. She had gotten carried away, misjudged the situation, made a spectacle of herself, had become an object of ridicule and now she had no place to hide. Instead, she hung her head in shame. As a feeling-state, shame involves the entire organism. Franz Alexander (1924) wrote:

> Shame is a reaction to feeling weak, ineffective, or inferior to others. The psychological reaction to shame is the opposite to that of guilt: it stimulates aggressiveness. To get rid of shame an individual has prove that he is not weak and can beat the person who shamed him. Shame is such a primitive reaction that even animals exhibit it; but guilt feelings can arise only after an individual has acquired a conscience, that is to say, after he has incorporated the moral values of his environment. (p. 370)

In other words, guilt is a superego function while shame is not. Incomprehensible as it may seem, the writer Primo Levi (1988) has always argued that the very fact of having been in Auschwitz, of not having rebelled, leaves a residue that will never go away: it is the shame of the victim, forever branded. Jean Amery (1980) made a similar observation with respect to torture. The victim *remains* tortured for the rest of his life. The experience of shame mobilizes the wish for the most primitive forms of retaliation, such as plucking out the eyes that were witness to that humiliation. Shame is perhaps the single most powerful human feeling-state. Nobody wants to die from guilt, but wanting to die from shame, wanting to disappear in the cracks of the sidewalk, is quite common. The novelist Salman Rushdie (1983) was inspired by a newspaper story to write his novel *Shame*. He states:

> Not so long ago, in the east end of London, a Pakistani father had murdered his only child, a daughter, because by making love to a white boy she had brought such dishonor upon her family that only her blood could wash away the stain. The tragedy was intensified by the father's enormous and obvious love for his butchered child, and by the beleaguered reluctance of his friends and relatives . . . to condemn his actions. Sorrowing, they told radio microphones and television cameras that they understood the man's point of view, and went on supporting him even when it turned out that the girl had never actually 'gone all the way' with her boyfriend. . . Between shame and shamelessness lies the axis upon which we turn; meteorological conditions at both of these poles are of the most extreme, ferocious type. Shamelessness, shame: the roots of violence. (pp. 123–4)

Being out of control, in and of itself, need not be shameful. Being *seen as* being out of control is immensely shameful and therefore enraging. While the out-of-control aspect of acute intoxication can be quite shameful, the imbiber is nevertheless thought of as being in control in the decision to drink in the first place and once again when sobered up. The same is not true for mental illness. W. C. Field's portrait of the drunk versus the crazy person captures the sentiment well: The drunk says: "I am drunk, and you are crazy. But tomorrow morning when we wake up, I will be sober but you will *still* be crazy."

While the frequent activation of the shame-rage cycle is by no means the exclusive property of patients suffering from bipolar disorders, it seems to be particularly common in that group of people, as well as in those populations which contain a large proportion of explosive personalities. It seems likely that in the case of the bipolar group some mood swings were operating early on in childhood. During the developmental stage of separation and individuation and specifically during what Margaret Mahler (1968) has called the practicing period, or subphase, the age-appropriate grandiosity and the age-appropriate exhibitionism were probably pronounced in these toddlers, since the zest which is normal for that age was fueled and intensified by varying degrees of mania, and the corresponding disappointments by depression. Consequently, the inevitable experiences of deflation must have been particularly painful. The toddler's love affair with the world encountered many dramatic rejections, failures, and rebuffs. Additionally, many of these patients remember being ridiculed, laughed at, and publicly humiliated or shamed by one or both parents. Typically, and not surprisingly, it is usually the parent who was also bipolar, who saw in the prancing toddler a mirror image of his own despised grandiose self which he now feels he has to persecute in the child. The rage generated by the shame-experience is a powerful emotional force which seeks retribution, revenge, and reparation. The alternative would be depression. In the comic strip *Peanuts*, Lucy induces Charlie time and again to kick off a football. However, just before he can do so she snatches the ball away and Charlie lands on his back, looking like a funny bug and feeling like a fool. Lucy's grandiosity remains intact. Charlie Brown, on the other hand, being a character in a mainstream American comic strip, cannot retaliate by beating her up nor can he resist the temptation to kick the ball, and consequently he ends up forever dejected and becomes, in his own words, "wishy-washy."

The experience of shame and humiliation during the stage of greatest narcissistic vulnerability leaves the child extremely sensitive to narcissistic injuries later in life. The expression of the corresponding rage can make a person feel foolish when confronted with its disproportionate nature. Shame and rage thus constitute a vicious cycle that feeds on itself. Sometimes the mere fact of being a patient can be experienced as humiliating and rage-provoking, and therefore demeaning. If to be diagnosed, and to be treated and medicated, spells being seen as being less than human, defective, and therefore unequal, the treatment is made vastly more complicated. Additionally, mania tends to stimulate grandiosity and, consequently, at times bizarre acting-out behavior which can be quite shameful and therefore enraging. As a result, chronic narcissistic rage is not an uncommon condition among bipolar patients and it requires a maximum of tact on the part of the therapist not to provoke or be provoked into a fight which is designed, from the patient's point of view, to indirectly repair real or imagined narcissistic wounds. If the patient begins a session with what during the Vietnam era was referred to by the military as a "defensive reaction strike," such as the statement "I did not come here to be sneered at," it can easily occupy the entire session and thereby avoid an unwanted discussion of the fact that the patient has yet again called and hung up the phone during office hours or paid his or her bill with a check that bounced. While understandable, such skirmishes are also quite counterproductive.

Perhaps the trickiest problem in this area is the question of free will versus self-responsibility. To what extent can we hold people responsible for the action they take or fail to take because of their affective impairment? To what extent should patients hold themselves accountable for their deeds? The first obstacle in the attempt to address this question is the difficulty many people have in distinguishing between, on the one hand, the concepts of guilt or fault, and on the other hand those of simple cause-and-effect relationships. The overtly depressed person *causes* many people to withdraw and to avoid the company of the depressive. As a logical explanation that would be acceptable to the depressive, but usually it is translated into the following: "It is all my own fault that nobody loves me and wants to be with me; I am guilty of making people feel uncomfortable." This translation into the realm of unworthiness is depressing in itself and it feeds the self-perpetuating cycle of a depressing lifestyle.

"If I cannot will myself to cheer up—or to simmer down—I deserve to be shunned" cannot become acceptable as a real challenge because the term "deserving" implies moral or ethical worth and it leaves no room for the biological component that may not always be under the patient's control. For example, the Internal Revenue Service, rightfully, takes an exceedingly dim view of the compulsive spending habits on the part of the manic patient if the mania is offered as an excuse for not having filed or paid taxes. Neurons, after all, do not move charge plates or write checks, only people can do that, and they will be held responsible for the consequences of their spending habits. The biological component only provides the impulses, not the direction, and it is the latter for which we assign responsibility. The impulse itself could be used just as easily to dig up an entire garden or to organize all dog owners into political action.

Liz, for example, at some point during her treatment, planned a trip to Europe. When we discussed the financial aspect of this plan, she showed me a budget for the six months preceding that trip which clearly indicated that the expense was one which she could readily afford. Since in the past she had frequently let her therapy bills accumulate and then pay them all at once, I was not overly concerned when that happened again. She firmly promised to pay before she left for Europe. Then she "forgot" to do this and then she was gone. In fact by the time she left she had already booked so many additions and extensions to her original trip that the cost of it added up to three times the amount she owed me. When she returned home she was not only broke but considerably in debt. Furthermore, during that particular summer I had also planned a somewhat exotic trip, similar to one Liz had taken a year before. All during her European trip, Liz vacillated between feelings of delight and pangs of guilt over the thought that by not paying me she might have caused me to give up my trip for lack of money. If that were to be the case, then she could continue to think of herself as that special person who had been the only one she knew to have been in that particular part of the world. Needless to say, her therapist was not amused and refused to accept the bipolar explanation as a sufficient excuse, particularly since she related her malevolent fantasy with such evident relish. While the mania provided the energy, it did not determine the use to which it was put. Hers were conscious, willful actions aimed at another person. There was indeed method to her madness, self-destructive, but governed by an infernal logic and it was built on the erroneous assumption that other people's financial affairs would be as chaotic as her own.

The problem of accountability obviously has as its corollary the question of control. If a person seems to be unable to control behavior, and if that behavior is deemed to be dangerous or injurious to either the person or to those around the person, hospitalization has to be considered. Aside from the question who is to decide what constitutes danger to self or others, obviously everything that has been said about medication and stigmatization applies to hospitalization at least doubly. Though there are data to support the contention that once a patient is hospitalized the chances for rehospitalization increase probably as much as fourfold, we do not know what the effect of the stigma is, as compared to other variables, such as severity of the disorder; but it seems reasonable to assume that it plays a considerable role unless it can be reframed.

Bernie, for example, never had to deal with the problem of stigmatization, because he defined his overnight stay at Bellevue Hospital as an emergency room treatment for an accident rather than as a hospitalization for mental illness. Since there was only an accident, there was no need to talk about it; the event became not exactly a secret, it was put in the "inactive" file. The issue of suicide, its prediction and prevention among patients suffering from affective disorder, poses a number of mostly insoluble theoretical, practical philosophical and ethical problems. With respect to hospitalization we have to weigh the negative effect of stigmatization and shame associated with institutionalization against the degree of suicidal danger. Should one ever take a chance? Should one allow some people to decide whether they want to live or die? What constitutes a "sound mind"? There are no clear-cut answers to any of these questions.

Predicting the probability for the frequency of suicides for groups of people is relatively easy. Among the total of 134 suicides committed in the year 1958 in St. Louis, Missouri, 94% were diagnosed as having suffered from psychiatric illness at the time of death. Of these, 47% were suffering from bipolar disorder, depressive phase, and 25% were alcoholics (Eli Robins, 1981). Similar studies were conducted for the populations of suicides during the years 1966–68 in West Sussex County in Great Britain, and for the years 1957–58 for those in Seattle, Washington. Robins, who analyzed the data, ranging over a 10-year span, concluded that the data clearly indicate that *in combination*, affective disorders, depressive phase, and alcoholism are the diagnoses predominantly associated with completed suicide, with a mean of 70% of the 324 suicides studied. Schizophrenia, on the other hand, accounted for only 5% of the overall sample. Furthermore, 73% of the subjects had sought some form of psychiatric help during their last year of life.

These statistics are probably representative for the country as a whole and as such quite depressing. However, in terms of prognosis for people suffering from affective disorder, they have to be understood in their demographic context: socioeconomic status, race, age, religion, and marital status. The populations examined in the three studies mentioned consist primarily of poor, unemployed, white, older, unattached or divorced males. In other words, an alienated, aged, disenfranchised group of people without social support systems and with limited access to *adequate* medical and psychiatric care. Put differently, the percentage of bipolar patients among successful suicides tells us nothing about the probability of suicide among bipolar patients unless we know a great many other things about them.

In general, women attempt suicide 10 times as often as do men. Men, on the other hand, succeed four times as often as do women, but men typically choose means that are failure-proof, such as guns; women tend to pick "softer," less reliable means, such as drugs. We also know that people who attempt suicide tend to try it again, until they either get effective help or until they are dead. But to predict suicidal risk for a particular patient is at times all but impossible.

Greg, for example, who came from a family where in each generation one male had died from suicide, at the age of 22, confided to his employer, a physician, that he feared the same as his own fate and therefore asked for psychiatric help. His boss made an appointment for him for the following day and assured Greg that he would make it through the night without trouble. At seven o'clock the following morning Greg went to the kitchen, took a small paring knife, and with it cut both his wrists and slit his throat from one side to the other. At that time he was renting a room with a family, who heard the sound of his falling, and rushed to his room, but there was no way for them to stem the rapid flow of blood and to save his life. The attack on himself had been too savage. In fact, it had been so ferocious that the coroner, a seasoned professional, after having viewed the body an hour later, asked for a solid shot of cognac. The immediate question that arose, of course, was why was he not hospitalized immediately? The only possible answer is, somebody made a judgment, and unfortunately that judgment turned out to have been wrong. To the best of everybody's knowledge this had been the first time Greg had asked for help. If fact, when he proudly showed his landlady how he had decorated his room, she asked him whether or not he knew that the only print he had hung in his room was of the painting that was on Vincent van Gogh's easel when he committed suicide; he merely indicated that he knew this. He clearly did not use that opportunity to ask for help, but it seems plausible that the fact that his father had killed himself while he was in the hospital apparently suggested to Greg that getting help is not necessarily helpful.

We cannot predict accurately who will succeed in committing suicide, and even if we feel reasonably certain, we cannot always prevent it. People who are determined to kill themselves will do so, no matter what. Even if they are conflicted about whether they want to live or die, they may not make that decision one way or the other. Instead they may feed their ambivalence by simply leaving that decision to chance. Typical examples are drinking and driving, drag-racing, visiting dangerous neighborhoods and starting fights, or, alternatively, failing to take action where action is indicated, such as seeking medical attention for serious illness or injuries, not getting the car fixed when neither steering wheel nor brakes function properly, or not getting out of the way when there is clear and present danger. If the result is death, it usually enters the police blotter as accidental death, accident, accidental overdose, or fatal mugging. However, such a tragic development is often the end product of a long process. Usually it involves a series of unsuccessful interactions between the family and the patient, the patient and a number of mental health professionals, or both. To a large extent, the degree to which these interactions can be improved is perhaps the best prognostic indicator of whether or not such unhappy outcomes will in fact occur.

In Chapter Two I mentioned a patient by the name of William, the man with the outsized appetites. His daughter, Paula, had been a fairly regular recreational user of heroin, which is in and of itself a fairly unhealthy habit. Additionally, however, this dramatically attractive young woman who always dressed for maximum sensual effect, usually bought her drugs in a high-crime area, late at night. Quite often she would do this while already high or under the influence of alcohol and in a car that can only be described as a death trap. Though one could look at her as someone who has primarily an addiction or substance-abuse problem, in addition to an infantile personality, that is also not the entire story. She comes, after all, from a family where in addition to assorted addictions, there is also a prevalence of bipolar disorders. Several years ago, Paula had undergone detoxification, but when it was to be followed by a six-month program of rehabilitation, she panicked and fled. Since she was over 21, legally she could do as she pleased, which included risking her life in the ways she did.

In order to have even half a chance to succeed with psychotherapeutic treatment, we decided to remove what we knew to
be the least of her problems, namely the biological component,
by putting her on Lithium. Since it was William, the father, who
was paying for it all, he had to be sold on that idea. Approaching
the subject was quite tricky, because it threatened to expose a
number of potentially taboo subjects: (1) The defective gene; this
concept was hinted at but given William's near attack of
apoplexy it was dropped immediately and never mentioned
again. (2) Addiction; while William had no problems acknowl-
edging that his sister and his daughter were "junkies," to suggest that either he himself or his sainted father might have had a
substance-abuse problem bordered on heresy. Paula's mother,
William's first wife, never failed to blame William to his face for
Paula's drug problems, taking visible pleasure in watching his
silent, and sometimes not-so-silent fury. She was sure that Paula
had "inherited" the problem and she never looked at the fact
that she was the one who forever bailed out Paula when she was
in financial trouble. Also, she never noticed when Paula nodded
out over the dinner table, she took it as a sign of fatigue due to
too much partying. Furthermore, William's second daughter
from his second marriage seemed also clearly troubled. Whether
she was merely shy and intimidated or whether she was mildly
depressed was also not to be questioned. Unless her behavior
could be blamed on her "crazy" mother, a recovered alcoholic,
the subject was not open to discussion. (3) Enabling; The interactive patterns that allow an individual to become addicted and
to stay addicted. In this case the subject had the potential for
exposing dangerous and explosive family secrets. For example,
William's third wife, Paula's stepmother, had taught Paula at the
age of fourteen how to freebase cocaine. Furthermore, Paula's
boyfriend, a married man, who supplied Paula with money to
keep herself and him supplied with drugs, was a business partner of William's. That meant that reporting him to the authorities, telling his wife, or simply knee-capping him in a back
alley would have had painful economic consequences. Addi-

tionally, given how the American legal code looks upon individual entrepreneurial gambling activities and bookmaking, there was a limit to which this family could risk any kind of legal exposure. What Paula's drug problems brought to the fore was the degree to which each and every member of that extended multigenerational "step- and steppes-step" patchwork quilt of a family was invested in protecting their own and other members' secrets. Exposing some of them would have meant jail for more than one of them, primarily, however, for the breadwinner of that extended clan. Had Paula's problems arisen earlier than they did, she would have had no chance for effective help from her family. But given the fact that William and his third wife, a former call girl and recovered heroin addict, had both been in psychotherapy, together with the fact that both were quintessentially decent and well-meaning human beings, the extended family could now be rounded up, some secrets could be exposed and dealt with, appropriate feelings of responsibility and regret felt and expressed, and the family could become Paula's safety net. Though Paula still has a drug problem, the family has extended enough vigilance, surveillance, and support to have vastly reduced the suicidal aspects of Paula's drug-taking behavior. What will happen eventually, only time will tell.

What this case illustrates so clearly is that the prognosis for patients with affective disorders depends to a large extent on the way in which the family comes to grips with the three S's—shame, stigma, and secrecy—and how the attitudes toward the subject can change over time. Ten years ago Paula had had total blackmailing power over her stepmother, William's third wife. Then she would have been terrified at the thought that William would learn about her freebasing cocaine and teaching his daughter to do the same. She would have feared that William might divorce her. Now, however, she freely admitted having done some things that were clearly destructive, thoughtless, and immature. But she can also point to the fact that she is no longer the same person she was then, that she is willing to assume some of the responsibilities of a stepmother. She genuinely regrets what she has done, and she is willing to make some reparations. Addiction in this family was seen as neither particularly stigmatizing nor particularly shameful, as long as it was viewed as a behavioral problem rather than a genetic impairment, and as long as the family icons remained untouched. Mental illness as a concept that could apply to any member of this family was unacceptable, while immaturity, neurosis, and addiction were sufficient as explanatory variables to account for most of their "crazy" behavior patterns. With respect to all of the family secrets, the exposure of some of them had been experienced as a breath of fresh air, while others are still taboo and probably will remain so for a long time to come.

It is estimated that in the U.S. about 40% of the people suffering from mood disorders never get any kind of treatment at all. While secrecy, shame, and stigma certainly account for a solid proportion of motives for not seeking help, cultural values, religion, ignorance, and social class also play a considerable role. For example, Puritanism and Christian Science, as systems of thought, both stress the nontherapeutic solution to all illness. Help can only come from either God or an individual's will and the determination to be strong, resilient, and to pull oneself up by one's own bootstraps. Additionally, the fear of being accused of malingering or self-indulgence keeps many older individuals from seeking professional help. The ignorance on the part of the general population about the treatment possibilities for affective disorders would be astounding if it could not be explained by the prevalence of irrational fears associated with mind-altering drugs and mental illness.

Social class and geographic location are also considerable handicaps towards getting proper psychiatric care. Outside of the large cities and depending on one's social class, medication to treat the "nerves" usually is restricted to minor tranquilizers, major tranquilizers, and sleeping pills.

Finally we have to mention that a small portion of patients suffering from affective disorders become what we call "career patients," i.e., people who define themselves primarily in terms of their impairment. This can happen in two ways. One, a patient simply gives up. One breakdown too many, too much work to start all over again, too much strain to pretend to feel cheerful when one is depressed, the discrepancy between one's achievement and that of peers has become too big, are all reasons to throw in the towel. Two, the family as a system accepts, welcomes, or needs a "sick" member. They can do this for countless reasons, none of which have anything to do with the actual problems of the family member elected. Some families need a black sheep, a substitute for a baby, a diversion from some other family dysfunction, a special person to indulge, an excuse not to socialize, or the need for a family secret which keeps them unique and separate from the rest of the world. The family dynamics in such instances are extremely powerful forces, because quite often it is the patient who holds the family together. On some level the patient knows this, and being now in fact impaired, breaking up the family would be tantamount to suicide.

For example, in one family I know, mother and son are forever wedded to each other. In a fit of rage the son either threatened to or actually did kill his father. The authorities as well as the rest of the family will never know what did happen. That particular secret will most likely follow them to their respective graves. In the meantime, however, they form a separate and very special family subgroup, one in which the son will never abandon his mother.

CHAPTER TEN

Case Material
Portraits Revisited

What keeps people happy and free from sadness and depression is a cluster of variables which, taken together, constitute what Sigmund Freud called "the ability to love and to work." We need to belong and we need to feel good about ourselves. Consequently people who have been given a psychiatric diagnosis have to first integrate that information into their ongoing biographies in such a way that their self-esteem and their sense of belonging is not diminished by that label. A diagnosis of an affective disorder usually also sheds a new and different light on the story of one's life, provides a benign explanation for some past events, and casts some doubts on some of one's own and other people's judgments. Additionally, it raises not a few questions with respect to the future. In that context the person/patient who grew up singled out as the "problem child," as "the crazy one," or the family scapegoat, faces the most difficult problems. They have struggled all their lives against parental invalidation and disqualification. After the diagnosis has been given, they tend to feel, at least initially, that their family's judgments have now been officially confirmed, that it was indeed the child who was always "crazy," i.e., wrong, guilty, the cause of the family's unhappiness. It takes some hard work sometimes for patients to realize that in terms of an understanding of a dysfunctional family dynamic they may indeed have been the only "sane" one, mood disorder notwithstanding.

If we compare the reactions on the part of the patients portrayed in Chapter two, we notice considerable differences between their reactions. Dorothy had the fewest problems, since from the *beginning*, she defined her illness as primarily medical—physical in origin. Her tearfulness was an understandable reaction to her physical impairment, and her corresponding inability to care for her family. Martha, who thought having a psychiatric problem far too shameful to even consider, knew nevertheless that in terms of her emotional stability something had gone very wrong. It never became clear to what extent she had been aware of her intermittent thought disorder, her dips into psychosis, since most of that experience had been "forgotten" by her. Once the depression lifted, she was able to either deny or to repress the details of that unhappy period. As far as she was concerned, there never was any psychiatric problem at all.

Bernie neatly and clearly distinguishes between "being neurotic" and "being mentally ill." He is clearly the former, and in that way, as far as he is concerned, he is no different from other creative and literary people. On the other hand, he was quite perturbed and felt rather ashamed about the public nature of his suicide attempt. It took some time until he reached the point at which he could feel genuine compassion for the refugee child who had never learned to ask for help. But taking antidepressant medication has not been a problem for him, first of all since he looks at the biological component as something that comes almost automatically with a Central European birth certificate and, secondly, his knowledge about the frequency of depression among literary families, such as the Hemingways, preceded his own depression. He never attended any AA meetings, since he does not think of himself as being any more of an alcoholic than other great writers, such as Faulkner, Hemingway, or Fitzgerald. In his judgment he is a normal depressive neurotic who, like so many other creative writers, at some point in their lives, drank too much. Consequently, he gave up drinking vodka and now sticks to wine and beer instead.

Of the patients discussed here, Mary had by far the most difficult time with the problem of integrating her diagnosis. It took her several years before she could say, "I am a manic-depressive" and still feel good about herself. She did that without having become a "career patient." She now knows that she has a chronic condition, that she will always need some medication, and that in addition to the coping skills she has already acquired, there are many more ways, which she has yet to learn, to help her control and to alleviate the more painful aspects of her bipolar disorder. At first, she could not get past the idea that perhaps underneath it all she really was some kind of "Son of Sam." "Without my medications, who would I be?" and "Which one is the real me?" are not questions that can be answered readily, if at all. Yes, who was that person who acted like a holy terror?

She has learned painfully that depending on her biochemical equilibrium, she can be either "well," i.e., feeling well (and being good) and thinking rationally; or she can be "off" which can mean either manic or depressed, but in her particular case that typically means thought-disordered. We have practiced almost like a litany the following evocation: When I feel this badly, I have three options: (1) I can increase my medication; (2) I can call my psychopharmacologist; or (3) I can walk into the emergency room of the nearest general hospital and be taken care of until I feel better; but *I do not have to go crazy and jump out a window*. She has never taken advantage of the third option, i.e. going to an emergency room, because, for one, she never felt bad enough to need it, but, two, because she knows that doing so would have been quite injurious to her self-esteem. The few times when she attended a manic-depressive support group, she was simply appalled by the casualness with which the other group members spoke about their numerous hospitalizations. Being as psychologically astute as she is, she clearly recognized how easy it can be to derive one's sense of specialness from having the "worst" case of mental illness and the most hospitalizations of all patients in all of recorded history. She also knows herself well enough not to ever want to tempt herself in that fashion. She has arrived at the following definition of herself as a depressive: Among patients suffering from bipolar disorders, and among those who have never been hospitalized, hers is the most serious and severe case. That is probably a fairly accurate assessment. Though it is at times still difficult for her, she has accepted that at times and in some instances she has to relinquish control. For example, her medication is not for her to decide. Her judgments regarding some specific professional, financial, or educational choices cannot always be trusted and therefore must be brought in line with the judgments of her therapists and the other health professionals involved in her care.

Liz resolved her problem in yet another way. While in terms of neurometric patterns, her EEG readings, the bipolar involvement is rather marginal, and since she has discovered that additionally she suffers from a host of learning disabilities, she has reframed her problem as being strictly neurological. She sees herself as a person with a medical handicap, and one who has been victimized by the psychiatric profession all her life. This alters her standing as a patient and as a citizen quite profoundly. She has been discriminated against by man and by nature. Therefore she should be entitled to have provisions made for her, so that the victim not be additionally victimized by the social institutions she now interacts with and needs.

For example, in her case, time limits, course load, and other restrictive rules of academic life should not apply to a person who is handicapped, i.e., impaired in her ability to read and to process information. Given this definition of the situation, she now made the physical rehabilitation and the remediation of her cognitive impairments her first priority. That project involved, besides a psychotherapist and a psychopharmacologist, a reading specialist, a cognitive psychologist, and a psychic. She explored and pursued all of those avenues while going to school and maintaining her private practice. She reasoned that if she went to school part-time she might become ineligible for financial assistance until such time as her status as a handicapped person was established. Given the fact that all those professional services which she required, together with some of the gadgets that were employed in her rehabilitation, put a considerable strain on her budget, her project of making herself over required quite an economic juggling act where soon the proverbial Peter had to be robbed to pay the proverbial Paul.

In terms of defining the work that psychotherapy, or other ways of adjusting to a diagnosis of depression, is supposed to accomplish, it may be helpful to recall the variables which singly or together constitute what is called the "final common pathway." Then we can examine how, in the case of each of the patients presented here, these variables interfered with the patient's ability to love and to work, in other words, to meet their affiliative needs and to regulate self-esteem. That comparison should suggest the treatment plan or what route to take if depressed people are to feel better. The variables are: (1) genetic vulnerability; (2) developmental events; (3) psychological stresses; (4) physiological stresses; and (5) personality or character traits.

In Mary's and Bernie's case, their understanding of the biogenetic component shed a very different light on the way they saw their parents, who had suffered from similar problems, but without the benefits of diagnosis and, consequently, treatment. It made sense to Bernie that his parents, whose circumstances had been quite difficult to begin with, lived the lives of recluses. One of the most important steps in his understanding of himself came when instead of only investigating the impact that his many losses in early life had had on his own development, he realized that while he thought he had lost his parents, they too had to adjust to what they believed to be the death of their only child. He had often wondered why he had no siblings. Now he began to suspect that they had simply never gotten over the imagined loss of Bernie and that therefore they did not feel equipped to risk another attachment, the loss of which they knew to be too devastating. He began to understand that what he experienced as "cardboard people," their two-dimensional qualities, were in fact the symptoms of a general and profound demoralization, one not too dissimilar to his own.

For Mary the problem was much more complicated. She had loved her father very deeply, even though his actions were those of a mean and terrifying tyrant, with entirely unpredictable rages and physical violence. But since there was no connection between her feelings of love for him and her experience of fear and hatred for this man, these emotions existed on parallel tracks, so to speak. The fact that she now had an explanation for his erratic behavior, instead of helping her, made it, at least initially, more difficult for her. Knowing the bipolar origins of his problems raised the possibility that she herself might be very much like her father; that she had inherited, along with the mania, also his despicable characteristics. Having been on the receiving end of his outbursts, she knew only too well how the victim feels. The thought that she might affect other people in the same or a similar way, that without her medications she could act as he did, was quite abhorrent to her. It took her almost two years before she understood that even though she might have very similar impulses, she nevertheless had also a well-developed conscience that would not permit her to act on her impulses for any length of time. While she, too, understands that desperation leads to desperate acts, some of them not particularly nice, that comprehension also is quite double-edged in her mind. But, when she finally understood the relationship between morality, cause, and effect, as well as responsibility, she presented me with that understanding in the form of a large and elaborate board game called "The Manic Game." It resembles Monopoly, but the only tokens used are *one* queen and half a dozen serfs (!). The entries depict the strategies of manic patients, such as, "Tell your therapist how terrific she is, and then threaten suicide" (move ahead three spaces), or "threaten to throw out all your medications and then call your mother" (move back five spaces). With that game, which takes its name from a serious research paper "Playing the Manic Game," published in the *Archives for General Psychiatry* (Janowsky, Leff, and Epstein, 1970), she handed me much more than just a piece of intellectual comprehension. This paper, which articulates and addresses some of the most enraging strategies of the acutely manic patient, does not always speak kindly in describing just how infuriating and frustrating these patients can be. It lists and discusses the following maneuvers as typical of this group of patients:

1. Manipulation of self-esteem of others: sensitivity to issues of self-esteem in others, with the increasing or lowering of another's self-esteem as a way of exerting interpersonal leverage. "Admire your therapist's skills, then cancel the next appointment without notice" (move ahead one space).

2. Perceptiveness to vulnerability and conflict: the ability to sense, reveal, and exploit areas of covert sensitivity in others. "Complain about group members to your therapist, but never tell them what you think" (move back one space).

3. Projection of responsibility: the ability to shift responsibility in such a way that others become responsible for the manic's actions. "Blame all your troubles on the fact that one day the group did not listen to you" (move ahead two spaces).

4. Progressive limit testing: the phenomenon whereby the manic extends the limits imposed on him, upping the ante. "Call your therapist 10 times per day, call again, and then hang up on her" (move ahead three spaces).

5. Alienating family members: the process by which the manic distances himself from his family (p.253). By putting her own behavior into this context, she has in fact admitted that much of it is in fact acting-out behavior and therefore subject to control. Calling it a game also makes it sound a lot less special and esoteric. Needless to say, the Manic Game has a permanent and honored position on the mantle of the fireplace in my office, where it serves as a handy reference.

Liz made it a point to talk to her family of origin about her diagnosis in order to make them aware of the fact that bipolar problems run in families and therefore could develop in any of their offspring. While she understands now that her father's explosiveness and his violence were in part rooted in biology, that understanding has not diminished her contempt for him in particular and for men in general. Because, she argues, only in a patriarchal, chauvinist society would such brutal behavior on the part of the "male head of household" be tolerated as acceptable behavior. While this is a reasonable argument, it additionally allows her to put her own rages and those of her father into two entirely different categories: hers are the reaction on the part of the oppressed while his represents the random violence of the oppressor. Hers are excusable, his are not.

Martha had defined herself primarily as a wife and as a mother. She also took considerable pride in her critical intelligence and in her knowledge of literature. Many of the people surrounding her experienced her intellectual standards as quite intimidating. Given the fact that she also had quite a sharp tongue, not too many people dared to enter her privacy, come too close or, violate one of her strictly defined boundaries. Her intimate confiding relationships were restricted to her family, to Rob, and to her parents. They constituted the intimate center of her life. Furthermore, on a level of intimacy which was one removed, i.e., warm but not confiding, there existed her and Rob's friends and the rest of the extended family. Finally, she knew a group of younger people, current or former employees of Rob's, who confided in her, but not the other way around. To them she was more of a respected mentor rather than a friend. In terms of meeting her affiliative needs and in supporting her self-esteem, the system was balanced; it worked well enough for her. However, losing the entire center of her intimate life within the span of a few years, together with the loss of her job-description as wife and mother, she was left with very little that could give her a sense of belonging, of being needed and feeling good about herself. She suspected that she might have to build an entirely new life for herself, but she knew no guidelines for such a daunting task. Ultimately, what it took was not a new life at all, but letting existing friendships be closer, become more intimate, and then to find work which she could be proud of. When I use the terms "intimate and confiding" in this context, I mean something quite simple and yet fundamental: We need someone on Monday who really wants to know how dinner went the previous Sunday, someone who worries about the dog's heat rash and who cares when the children fail to call. In other words, we need someone with whom we can share the stuff of everyday life, even if it is only over the phone or by letter. Martha had been that confiding "other" for her own parents, and she found it difficult to accept that her own children could not or would not do likewise. They rightly sensed that in this instance the job of mothering the mother was a task they were not equipped to handle in the way she wanted it. Since she also knew clearly that she did not want to fall in love again and to remarry, that meant that she had to learn to relate to nonfamily members, i.e., friends, in ways that satisfied her needs for closeness, and at the same time not to come too close for comfort. In order to accomplish this she had to become quite a bit more tolerant of other people's tastes and intellectual limitations and shortcomings. This she did; she developed several close friendships and, in addition, she retained and expanded the circle of younger people who, as adults, continued to confide in her and to help her with some of the practical problems in her life, such as moving the heavy geranium pots. In her search for work she was very lucky, in that she found steady freelance editorial work, tailor-made for her particular talents, appreciative of her versatility and her critical judgments and flexible enough to suit her mobility. She took great pride in her work and she liked the fact that she was indeed indispensable.

Once her depression lifted, her health improved dramatically; she had replacement surgery, and she is again quite mobile. On the whole, she is probably more contented than she has ever been. She has managed successfully *not* to give up previous satisfactions, but has learned to fill them differently, in ways that are commensurate with her changed circumstances. For example, she no longer mourns the dog that her lack of mobility prevents her from keeping. Instead she is now as crazy about her three cats as she had been about the dog.

Strictly speaking, Bernie did not really lose anything real and concrete. Receiving that rejection letter from the editor he so admired was like surrendering the flag to a country he never possessed. To a large extent, Bernie had always lived in a world of dreams and of symbols. He did not really belong anywhere. He was, naturally, bilingual, but without being truly at home in either language. His fragile self-esteem rested on unrealized potential as well as on a great deal of repressed grandiosity. He had no immediate family and he barely knew his parents. He had never been deeply in love with any woman and he had only a few close friends. Underneath that affable persona there was a rather haughty, contemptuous, but frightened self, one that was lonely and disconnected from people. What Bernie needed immediately after his suicide attempt was, in addition to antidepressant medication, a project to immerse himself in. The psychiatrist at the hospital had put Bernie on a tricyclic antidepressant which worked well for him. I then challenged him to write his family history. Fortunately, at that time he had some money saved up, and he was therefore able to make several trips to Florida in order to get to know his parents for the first time and to collect the oral history of the clan. Eventually, he took several trips to Austria, where he researched his family history, met relatives he never knew existed, and could see himself as part of an extended family, with a history, traditions, location, and continuity. He also rediscovered the German language as his true mother tongue, one in which feelings and emotions are irrevocably tied to their symbolic representations. For example, when we recall particularly shameful events of early childhood, and do so in a foreign language, no matter how familiar, we only tell the facts; we do not feel or convey the feelings attached to them. They reside in the language in which they originally took place. Not surprisingly, Bernie discovered that he is also two different kinds of writer, depending on which language he writes in. In a similar way he can now also be two different kinds of patients. The project soon took on a life of its own, since after two years he managed to combine it with a job as a correspondent for an Austrian literary magazine. In his new incarnation as a writer, researcher, correspondent, he felt that his "real" life was still in limbo, suspended, and had yet to begin. He still depended on the dream of writing the "Great American (or German) Novel," in order to feel good about himself. In the meantime, however, earning a living as a journalist was good enough. By spending almost a third of his time on the continent, his ambivalence towards all commitments, which in the past he had played out through inactivity and passivity, he now had a chance to play out actively. By traveling as much as he did, it made indeed no sense to fill or defrost a refrigerator in either country. For several years the largest number of consecutive therapy sessions that he managed to keep was 20. For that reason I could also not put him into one of my ongoing therapy groups. If I had put him into one, he would not have been able to form any lasting attachments for two reasons. One, he was away too much but, two, the literary snob in him had to be toned down first for group work to be productive. He had to learn the difference between a PEN meeting and therapeutic work in a group setting. Once he had become a journalist, something qualitatively different from driving a cab, his "work" was a little too close in nature to the activity that would have produced the dream, namely writing. He had to distance himself from possible misidentification. What emerged was a considerable amount of hitherto repressed, unbridled grandiosity; in fact he took great pride in being "a contemptuous snobby pain," as he called it, who was blissfully unaware of how his view of people might affect the possibility of future friendships. Along with the grandiosity there also emerged a healthy measure of rage—

anger at a world that had deprived him of a homeland and a childhood. The Great Novel had become his homeland instead, the one country that nobody could take away from him. The anger that emerged he found quite frightening, so much so that several times during that period of treatment he was tempted to run away from it all. He seriously considered moving to Austria, where he could resume therapy "in Vienna where it had, after all, all begun."

For Bernie to recover from his depression, he had to truly enter and settle into *one* country, derive sufficient amounts of satisfaction from the work he is doing *now,* not at some future point, and to accept the fact that there will never be a magical love, springing from some mythical object, but that the human relationships already in existence can be made more rewarding and considerably more intimate. Finally, he has to make peace with the fact that the life he has is the only one he will ever have and, what is more, that the childhood he did not have cannot ever be restored to him. For that to take place, he had to first mourn all the years that he wasted, living in suspended anima-tion, in anticipation of the return of a paradise he had lost some 50-plus years ago in Vienna. Only then could he begin to make peace with the life he actually inhabits and not to make happi-ness contingent on writing the great masterpiece. To the degree that he is learning to accept himself, as is, he can also be more tolerant and accepting of others and not demand that they be geniuses in order to be acceptable as intimates.

Bernie's stays in New York have become progressively long-er, he recently even acquired a large cactus for his apartment here, in other words, a plant that requires water every eight weeks, but not so often as to make him feel that he is tied down. Bernie, who does a great deal of his therapeutic work by writing me letters, recently indicated that he feels that when he reaches the point where he can write one entire letter without switching languages even once, he might then be able to settle down. He still does not say where, though. While he no longer has the "object constancy" appropriate for a flight attendant, he also has not yet developed a genuine desire to give up his assorted transatlantic escape hatches. The irony has not escaped him entirely that the man who for almost 20 years never left Greenwich Village except to drive his cab, now has trouble spending more than a day below 14th Street. Besides helping him avoid a commitment to either a specific identity, place, or particular line of work, his traveling has also had another function: it avoids temptation. After all, he knows from his own experience only too well how easy it is to settle in some place, not really live, not think about the future concretely, but to live inside one's own head in the anticipation of a glorious future. He knows; he did it for almost two decades. His being constantly on the move is, in a way, almost counterphobic. Eight months ago, Bernie began to decrease his medication and, two months ago, he discontinued it altogether. He is now assuming the responsibility for maintaining his moods without pharmacological help.

Mary has had the extremely difficult task of putting her entire life back together and to integrate into it an illness that in her case is very difficult to manage and to control. She had to accomplish this without the relative financial security she had enjoyed previously. For the first 18 months of her breakdown, all she could do was to manage her job in some fashion, take just one college course per semester, and devote the rest of her energy to concentrating on adjusting to her medications, to have her drug composition and relative dosage adjusted for her—finetuned to her needs, as it is so elegantly called—a term that neglects to mention that the process can be rather strenuous for the patient concerned—and to stay out of a mental hospital.

Only after she was stabilized pharmacologically could she move from damage control to the job of reconstruction. That meant a number of things. After her catastrophic venture into real estate, which had cost her not only all her inherited money, but also her rent-controlled apartment, she had to find a new place to stay. In addition, she had to find a new job, one where she could work full-time, which in the job she then had was not possible. She planned on coming back to her old therapy group, and she knew that she also had to build a social support system and to plan for a life as free from stress as can ever be possible when one lives in New York City. The hardest part by far was coming to grips with the problem of stigmatization. This task could not be delayed. There was a specific and compelling reason, namely her wish to rejoin her therapy group. During her two-year absence a new member had joined the group. Unfortunately, one day when Mary had had a particularly violent attack of mania, and therefore rang my office bell incessantly, she effectively ended a session for that particular patient who then had to be rescheduled. Consequently, the two of them met in the hall, they saw each other while coming and going, and neither one of them, naturally, forgot. Before returning to her group she had to deal with the shame of having been seen entirely out of control, acting like a deranged person instead of a normal neurotic. During her absence from group Mary had gone to great lengths to keep in regular contact with all members. She had also done everything within her power to conceal from them the depth of her disturbance. This she succeeded in to an astonishing degree. After she was gone for only six months, the group could not understand why I did not invite her back sooner. They all felt that "she was doing just fine." Mary had been quite proud of that fact and she was therefore extremely distressed at the thought that there would now be *one* person in the room who knew better—who had seen her at her worst. Of all the tasks she had to face, this was by far the most difficult. After she had gotten over her initial rage at me for having put that particular patient into *her* group, the one to which I knew she would eventually return, she had to then deal with the painful reality that having been out of control does not confer special privileges; that regardless of how troubled she might be, I would continue to honor my obligations to my other patients. She experienced my action as a form of punishment for bad behavior, and as such, profoundly unjust. "I could not help myself at that time," she argued and we had to argue the contention time and again, that outside of a mental hospital nobody could ever protect her from the social consequences of her own actions. What made this particularly difficult to accept and to work through was the fact that after her excursion into real estate, Mary's boss had employed his own attorney to rescue Mary from the most serious consequences of her manic grandiosity. Though the adventure cost her dearly, the lesson that the concept of "diminished responsibility" and "not of sound mind" could be used in her favor had indeed sunk in. It also confused her considerably. The idea that in court she should *not* appear reasonable and sane, but that in all other situations she should, was still too difficult to comprehend. The lighthearted suggestion that she would not hurt her own case in the least if she bit the judge or growled at the district attorney she did not see as being sensible. She also did not think it the least bit funny. All she could think of was how to impress the judge with what a responsible and law-abiding citizen she was. Being, at that time, unable to remember always the difference between civil and criminal proceedings, she only thought of a judge as somebody who metes out punishment and puts people in jail. All that took some doing to sort out.

After these legal problems had been settled, Mary could begin to look for a new place, move into it, and start looking for a new job, since her boss did not at that time need another full-time person. He did, however, recommend her to a colleague. The transition into her new position went surprisingly smoothly.

The therapeutic task, once she had settled in a new job and a new apartment was to help her to muster enough motivation to want to get better. The notion that someone should need help in finding the amount of motivation that is sufficient for recovery should not be surprising, because getting better usually means giving up the special privileges that are associated with the role of the sick person in our society, such as attention, diminished responsibility, specialness, etc., all the things that give us back—temporarily, at least—the "tyranny of infancy," when we can do no wrong. What had to be addressed first was the existential question, "What would the world offer her in return for getting better?" I had no answers. Mary, like all of us, had to find the answer within herself. In her case it happened at first almost indirectly. Initially, attending some of the meetings of a manic-depressive support group accomplished almost the opposite of its intended purpose. The last thing Mary wanted to be was "one of them." She did not like the picture of a group of people for whom the mood disorder was so central to their lives and to their identity that all other more rewarding goals were subordinated to it and thereby lost their intrinsic meaning. Knowing that she had to choose between living by the rules of the subculture of the mentally ill and those of the "normal majority," she liked the idea of belonging to the majority better, even though she has to compete in it with a considerable handicap. Making this decision was particularly difficult for Mary, since three of her fellow group members are already psychotherapists who have mostly completed their education, while her own academic plans suffered a serious setback. For the time being, she has to actually enjoy her job as such, instead of seeing it as merely a means towards an end. Instead of it being just something she does that pays her rent while she is going to school, she has to actually appreciate the good work that she is in fact producing. While she is continuing her education and doing it as well as ever, the time perspective, i.e., the projected length of time required to finish it, has changed a bit.

In order better to adjust to the fundamental injustice that is inherent in all serious illness, Mary did some volunteer work with AIDS patients. That meant two things. One, Mary was grateful for being alive; and, two, she realized that she was doing some therapeutic work after all. However, after having lived through three deaths in rapid succession, Mary decided that working with the terminally ill was too stressful for her. Instead she is now planning to continue doing volunteer work, but to do so in the context of some "big sister" program. She has found that in her capacity for compassion and for the intuitive understanding of other people's troubles, the experience of having a bipolar disorder has also given her something special in a very healthy and positive way. She now knows that she knows things that healthy people will never know. At this point she feels that the suggestion to organize a support group with a telephone hot-line for people who have had manic-depressive illness but who have never been hospitalized, is still too difficult a project, too intimidating a task, even though she is perfectly aware of the fact of how much it is needed for people with problems similar to hers. The need for an ear, is in this case, not something to be regulated by specific days and particular hours, but *whenever* mania threatens to take over, or whenever an acute change of mood occurs. In other words, a phone is imperative the *very* moment the mood switch hits.

In some way or another, she will undoubtedly do something of that kind. Eventually she will want to utilize her experience and to put it to good use where it is needed. Among other reasons for my thinking this way is the fact that she so readily gave her permission to utilize her case history, warts and all, for this book. She did so for the simple reason that she assumes that it might possibly help people who either have or who treat affective disorders. From the very beginning of her breakdown she kept looking for something that would make her painful experience not worthwhile—nothing could do that—but at least give it a raison d'être. Maybe an active involvement such as a support group for fellow sufferers will be what is most suitable for her.

Liz, after having reframed her problem along strictly neurological lines, then found herself unable to meet the demands of graduate school, not for lack of intelligence or hard work, but for reasons having to do with the way she reads and the ways in which she processes and reproduces information. This unfortunate discovery has reactivated her most tender spots in terms of feeling shame, namely the fear of being thought of as stupid, as being too grandiose in terms of academic achievement and social mobility. Consequently it was of vital importance to her that every person she came in contact with was indeed convinced that she was *physically* handicapped and therefore in need of rehabilitation. However, even when nobody questioned her assertions, she was not at all convinced that we told her what we really thought. "Prove that you don't distrust me and what I say" is a demand that can never be met. So she continued to suspect that we all humored her in order to keep her as a patient or client because we needed her money. Her fear of being talked about, even laughed at, behind her back was so intense that she could not tolerate the thought that the various professionals who were working on her head, i.e., her psyche, her mind, her brain, and her study habits should be allowed to talk to each other. Though she knew that for reasons of professional courtesy alone, there had to be at least initially some communication between them, particularly since, with the exception of the psychic, her therapist had made all the referrals, she insisted on hearing each and every word spoken between them, probing for inconsistencies and inaccuracies, suspecting misrepresentations or vilification, and invariably finding at least one instance to confirm her suspicions. Additionally, her need to control and to manipulate the responses of others, or rather the responses she would have liked to have gotten, to manipulate the people trying to help her, was so powerful that she forever traded the judgments of one in opposition to those of another. Obviously, such an arrangement seldom works. For example, statements to her psychotherapist to the effect that her cognitive psychologist had informed her that the reason she could never balance her checkbook was the result of her learning disability—implying that none of it had been her fault—is designed to arouse suspicion and distrust in either the patient's motives or, alternatively, the intelligence, the integrity, and the competence of the other professionals involved.

The way the system was set up, the way Liz worked and manipulated it, was designed to fail, and to fail her in what she wanted the most: to be respected and to accomplish those goals which she thought would permanently restore her self-esteem.

Going to graduate school initially was designed to legitimize her professionally and to gain access to legitimate insurance reimbursements. Towards that end, a Master of Social Work degree (MSW) would have been perfectly sufficient. In fact, Liz herself found a program designed specifically for people in her position. It gives field work credits for clinical work done while the student is in school; all the classes required for graduation can be taken at night, on weekends, during the summer, or any combination thereof. It would have taken Liz no more than two years to complete the program. However, her grandiosity did not allow her to be "yet another undereducated social worker." Only the title Doctor of Philosophy would satisfy her. This complicated matters considerably. First of all, to get admitted into any Ph.D. program requires that the applicant take the Graduate Record Examination (GRE). Knowing from past experience how poorly she performs on standardized tests, Liz had to take a year out just to get tutoring in taking the GRE's. She did that, and she did well in them, though not well enough to get admitted into a clinical psychology program, which are notoriously hard to get into. Instead, she entered a psychology program which, in terms of her interests, was very exciting, but would not entitle the graduate to receive insurance reimbursements in New York State. Even the suggestion that she might be better off pursuing a Psy.D. (Doctor of Psychotherapy) program, which would have given her both, namely the title doctor and access to health insurance reimbursements, was rejected by Liz as not scholarly enough.

To complicate matters even further, after several months of being treated by three or four different professionals, she knew that soon she would be unable to pay for it all. Consequently, a considerable amount of time and energy now had to be devoted to the problem of how to stall whom for how much when she tried to negotiate her balance on her bills. She explained that just recently, due to her learning disability and her bipolar disorder, her private practice had shrunk considerably, and therefore her income. This last rationalization was particularly unfortunate. In reality it had been her disassociation from that radical lesbian therapy group that had cut her off from a considerable source of patient referrals, which was responsible for her lack of patients. After all, her learning disabilities and her affective disorder had been a constant in her life, while the determination to earn a living honestly was not. By explaining the state of professional affairs in that way to herself and to others, she effectively deprived herself of enjoying what should have been a genuine sense of pride, since it had been a demonstration of a newfound sense of integrity.

When Liz's psychotherapy bills exceeded the amount permissible, she decided to take a leave of absence in order to catch up financially. In the meantime she continues to see her psychopharmacologist, she attends a remedial reading program, and she is attempting to negotiate a graduate program that is commensurate with her disabilities.

Despite the premature and unfortunate interruption, the treatment in this instance has been quite successful in that her bipolar disorder has finally been detected and brought under pharmacological control. Additionally, Liz has gained at least a foothold in the professional middle class she so much wanted to be a part of. She has learned a great deal about what constitutes polite and appropriate behavior, proper outward appearance, she has a full set of new teeth, she has ongoing relationships with other people, and she owns a much beloved dog.

Her basic characterological problems have been touched on, but so far they have been too deeply ingrained and too interwoven with her coping skills to yield significantly to psychotherapeutic intervention. While in the past she took great pride in the ingenuity of her dishonest adventures, she has at least reached the point where she would prefer it if she could afford to get things honestly. Given the fact that this is not possible, she continues mostly in her old ways. But now she does so with at least a twinge of guilt.

In terms of her ability to love and to work, Liz is infinitely more connected to people than she was before. She has postponed the goal of "being in a relationship" until such time as she is "well" psychologically and until she has completed her graduate work. What that means is that almost all sources of satisfaction and self-esteem lie in the future. They are anticipated, but not yet a reality. In addition, she lives with a low-level terror of being "found out." She lives with the constant fear that she might either come upon a task she cannot master or of being tripped up by her past. Her various aliases, her misrepresentations of herself, unpaid debts and unmet legal obligations, all provide her life with excitement, but with not much peace of mind. Until she really mops up after herself, she cannot be sure of the fact that when she finishes school she will be able really to enjoy the fruits of her labor. Only time will tell whether Liz will meet the challenge. I hope she does.

Postscript
Behavioral Medicine

When this book was first conceived, the last chapter was tentatively titled "Applications of the Techniques of Behavioral Medicine for the Treatment of Mood Disorders." This choice of subject matter was not due to the fact that I knew of any such research, it merely seemed self-evident that it should exist. After all, behavioral medicine has utilized the mind to influence a large variety of physical organs, of which, theoretically, at least, the brain should be one. Therefore it did seem likely that my ignorance could be cured by a trip to the library or by questioning people working in either of the three subspecialties involved.

To my great surprise that assumption turned out to be wrong. There are no specific data of any significance. While everybody I have spoken to has indeed agreed that mine was a perfectly logical assumption, nobody has been able to tell why this omission exists. This holds true for biopsychiatrists as well as for psychologists specializing in techniques such as hypnosis, biofeedback, acupuncture, imaging, and the like, and it also holds true for researchers in behavioral medicine.

While there are some treatises in pop psychology which suggest that the reader picture him or herself as being already happy, slim, popular, or whatever, utilizing the power of self-hypnosis and of autosuggestion, both of which are undoubtedly beneficial, the scientific literature is silent on the subject.

In the course of the last decade or two, behavioral medicine has moved from the realm of the counterculture, or that of the New Age fringe into the domain of respectable mainstream medicine. It is estimated that approximately 400 medical schools in the U.S. offer some basic training in this specialty. When President Nixon visited China in 1972, James Reston, who covered the presidential trip for the *New York Times*, was stricken by appendicitis. He was operated on by Chinese doctors using conventional medicine. During the postoperative period, however, he developed severe pains, which his doctors treated with acupuncture. The news of Mr. Reston's experience was flashed around the world, and Western doctors began to take a very hard look at a practice they had so long ignored.

Pain research has devoted a great deal of attention to its transmission from site to brain. Three possible sites of intervention, or pain interception, have been examined. First, there is the location of the trauma itself, the wound or burn, where the chemicals prostaglandin and bradykinin are released, which then send a message to the brain. It travels along the sensory nervous system from the damaged tissue to the dorsal horn of the spinal column where various neurotransmitters are released. Those in turn relay the pain sensation to the thalamus and other specialized sensory centers in the brain. During the second or two when the pain message is in transit, it is *merely* a potential, not yet a reality. It would *remain* a potential if, at some point along the line, this message could be intercepted. The observation of such a phenomenon was particularly striking during World War II when U.S. army physicians, basing their prediction of need on civilian experience had accumulated a vast reserve of morphine. However, field surgeons were quite surprised subsequently to see men with shattered limbs, severe internal injuries, and horrible burns, acting as if they felt no pain at all, talking calmly and refusing narcotics. Meanwhile it took several decades until the discovery of the putative pain-modulating agents, namely the now-famous natural morphinelike substances (endorphins) produced by the brain. In situations of extreme stress, such as a serious injury, they can temporarily flood the pain receptors of the brain. Subsequent research has shown that the endorphins are produced in numerous sites or organs of the body and that they are involved in a large variety of protective and/or healing mechanisms of the organism. Most importantly, they influence the functions of the immune system.

There is mounting evidence that such states as loneliness, bereavement, and chronic stress, may affect the immune system. In addition, the *combined* presence of subclinical or clinical depression and of social isolation, which are often related, increases the risk for cardiac problems in men as much as tenfold. How does that happen? Obviously, bereavement, beliefs, how we feel about ourselves, the nature of our relationships with other people, and our position in the world are not directly connected to the heart. Livers, stomachs, and spleens do not apparently register grief, feel shame, or suffer from grief. Only the brain seems able to do that. The brain, however, through extensive networks of nerve and humoral connections between the thymus, spleen, bone marrow, and lymph nodes, can direct the immune system. Furthermore, the cells in the immune system appear to be equipped to respond to chemical signals from the central nervous system. Receptors for a variety of chemical messengers, such as catecholamine, prostaglandin, growth hormone, sex hormones, serotonin, and endorphins have been found on the surface of lymphocytes, one of the blood cells involved in warding off disease. Alternatively, major psychological upsets, such as being fired from a much coveted job, or a messy divorce, result in the release of several powerful neurohormones, including catecholamine, corticosteroids, and endorphins. These, in turn, can alter immune function.

The reverse relationship has also been suggested, namely the positive effect of hypnosis and imaging on the functioning of the immune system. People told under hypnosis to visualize their white blood cells as "powerful sharks" swimming through the bloodstream, and attacking weak, confused germs, seemed to show increased immune function and a rise in the number of lymphocytes. Being connected, caring for, in general, also seems to have a beneficial impact on the immune system, even if it is only caring for a pet or a plant. Going further, McClelland has shown that merely viewing a film about Mother Theresa tending to the sick and the dying in Calcutta, seemingly increased immune function, even among subjects who disliked Mother Theresa. While these findings are regarded as somewhat controversial, evolutionary biology suggests that they may not be too far off the mark. The inclination towards caring for is a trait which is useful for the group and therefore should evoke a positive response. In animal herds, overcrowding results in increased death rates, even if food supplies are adequate, indicating that there are some regulatory mechanisms in animals that respond to the needs of the group as a whole, as, for example, in this instance of the need for more space. In addition, actuary tables indicate that individuals who are no longer part of a viable social unit, such as a family, have a lowered resistance towards disease.

On the other hand, any strong connection or commitment to a group results in improved resistance, which makes sense in evolutionary terms, since an individual connected to the group is more valuable to the social unit's survival than one who is not. Endorphins seem to be implicated in a multitude of functions, not only in pain modulation, but in a number of mood-stabilizing phenomena as well, such as the runner's "high" and the runner's "calm." They also appear to be involved in the regulation of appetite and food cravings, laughter, tears, the thrill associated with intense pleasure mixed with danger, the regulation of hormone cycles, particularly during puberty and childbirth, and a host of others. The tenfold drop in endorphine levels from their peak within 24 hours after delivery greatly contributes to the "baby blues" or to the more severe forms, i.e., postpartum depression. In Chapter Seven I mentioned Reiser's concept of major psychoses representing stress disorders with the brain as the principal target. It also begs the question whether or not, for example, the benefits of biofeedback which have been demonstrated beyond reasonable doubt to mediate the impact of stress on the cardiovascular system, the digestive system, and the pulmonary system, would not also benefit the brain in moderating the deleterious effects of stress. Yet L. Rossi, who has claimed that hypnosis can change molecules even on the genetic level, strangely enough has not included affective disorders or the major psychoses in his discussion.

While, clearly, the potential for the application of the methods developed by behavioral medicine for the treatment of mood disorders is purely speculative on my part, my admittedly unsystematic survey among colleagues working in these subspecialties, asking them as to whether or not these speculations are biologically possible or impossible, has not yielded a single definitive answer one way or the other. While anybody familiar with the subject of depression would not expect to discover any methods that would revolutionize the treatment of these disorders—such as finding a behavioral alternative to Lithium treatment—it still looks like an avenue well worth pursuing.

However, to the extent that the thinking about the subject is no longer influenced by the presence of a mythical mind/brain dichotomy, the therapeutic integration of biopsychosocial factors will undoubtedly follow the conceptual one.

References

Ainsworth, M. D. S., Blehar, M. C., Waters, E., & Wall, S. *Patterns of attachment*. Hillsdale, NJ: Erlbaum, 1978.

Akiskal, H. S., & McKinney, W. T. Depressive disorders: Towards a unified hypothesis. *Science*, 1973, *182*, 20–29.

Akiskal, H. S., & McKinney, W. T. Overview of recent research in depression: Integration of ten conceptual models into a comprehensive clinical frame. *Archives of General Psychiatry*, 1975, *32*, 285–305.

Akiskal, H. S., Hirshfeld, R. M. A., & Yerevanian, B. I. The relationship of personality to affective disorders: A critical review. *Archives General Psychiatry*, 1983, *40*, 801–810.

Akiskal, H. S., King, D., & Scott-Strauss, A. Chronic depression, Part I. *Journal of Affective Disorders*, 1981, *3*, 297–315.

Alexander, F. *The history of psychiatry*. New York: New American Library, 1966.

American Psychiatric Association. *DSM-III-R: The diagnostic and statistical manual of mental disorders* (3rd ed.). Washington DC: American Psychiatric Association, 1987.

Améry, J. *At the mind's limits: Contemplations by a survivor of Auschwitz and its realities*. Bloomington: Indiana University Press, 1980.

Andreasen, N. C. *The broken brain*. New York: Harper & Row, 1984.

Anehensel, C. S., & Stone, J. D. Stress and depression: A test of the buffering model of social support. *Archives of General Psychiatry*, 1982, *39*, 1392–1396.

Anthony, E. J., & Benedek, T. *Depression and human existence.* Boston: Little, Brown, 1975.

Angst, J. *Zur aetiologie und nosologie endogener depressiver psychosen.* Berlin: Springer Verlag, 1966.

Arieti, S., & Bemporad, J. *Severe and mild depression: The psychotherapeutic approach.* New York: Basic Books, 1978.

Asberg, M., Traskam, L., & Thoren, P. 5-HIAA in cerebrospinal fluid: A biochemical suicide predictor? *Archives of General Psychiatry,* 1976, *33,* 1193–1197.

Atwood, G. E., & Stolorow, R. D. *Structures of subjectivity.* Hillsdale, NJ: The Analytic Press, 1984.

Ayd, F. J. *Recognizing the depressed patient.* New York: Grune and Stratton, 1961.

Bacciagaluppi, M. Some remarks on the Oedipus complex from an ethological point of view. *Journal of the American Academy of Psychoanalysis,* 1984, *12*(4), 471–490.

Bacciagaluppi, M., & Bacciagaluppi, M. The relevance of ethology to interpersonal psychodynamics and to wider social issues. *Journal of the American Academy of Psychoanalysis,* 1982, *10*(1), 85–111.

Baldessarini, R. *Biomedical aspects of depression and its treatment.* Washington, DC: American Psychiatric Association Press, 1983.

Balint, M. *The basic fault: Therapeutic aspects of regression.* New York: Bruner Mazel, 1968.

Balint, M. *Primary love and psychoanalytic technique.* New York: Liveright, 1953.

Bartlett, E. S., & Izard, C. E. A. A dimensional and discrete emotions investigation of the subjective experience of emotion. In Izard, C. E. A. (Ed.), *A new analysis of anxiety and depression.* New York: Academic Press, 1972.

Basch, M. F. *Understanding psychotherapy.* New York: Basic Books, 1988.

Beck, A. T. *Depression: Clinical, experimental and theoretical aspects.* New York: Harper & Row, 1969.

Becker, E. *The birth and death of meaning.* New York: The Free Press, 1962.

Becker, E. *The revolution in psychiatry.* New York: The Free Press, 1964.

Becker, E. Mill's social psychology and the great historical convergence on the problem of alienation. In I. L. Horowitz (Ed.), *The new sociology.* New York: Oxford University Press, 1965.

Bell, R. M. *Holy anorexia.* Chicago, IL: University of Chicago Press, 1985.

Bellack, A. S., Hersen, M., & Himmelhoch, J. W. A comparison of social skills training, pharmacotherapy and psychotherapy for depression. *Behavioral Research Therapy,* 1983, *21,* 101–107.

Berger, P. A., & Brodie, K. H. (Eds.). *American handbook of psychiatry, Vol. VIII.* New York: Basic Books, 1986.

Bloch, D. *So the witch won't eat me: Fantasy and the child's fear of infanticide.* Boston: Houghton Mifflin, 1979.

Bloom Feshbach, J., & Bloom Feshbach, S. *The psychology of separation and loss.* San Francisco, CA: Jossey-Bass, 1987.

Bellack, A. S., Hersen, M., & Himmelhoch, J. M. Social skills training, pharmacotherapy and psychotherapy for unipolar depression. *American Journal of Psychiatry,* 1981, *138,* 1562–1567.

Bemporad, J. New views on the depressive character. In Arieti, S. (Ed.), *The world biennial of psychiatry and psychotherapy* (Vol. I). New York: Basic Books, 1970.

Berger, P., & Luckmann, T. *The social construction of reality.* New York: Doubleday Anchor, 1967.

Bowlby, J. *Attachment and loss (Vol. I).* New York: Basic Books, 1969.

Bowlby, J. *Attachment and loss (Vol. II). Separation, anxiety and anger.* New York: Basic Books, 1973.

Bowlby, J. *A secure base.* New York: Basic Books, 1988.

Breger, L. *From instinct to identity: The development of personality.* Englewood Cliffs, NJ: Prentice Hall, 1974.

Brownmiller, S. *Against our will: Men, women, and rape.* New York: Simon & Schuster, 1975.

Briscoe, C. W., Smith, J. B., Robins, E., Marten, S. & Gaskin, F. Divorce and psychiatric disease. *Archives of General Psychiatry,* 1973, *29,* 119–125.

Briscoe, C. W., & Smith, J. B. Depression in bereavement and divorce. *Archives General Psychiatry,* 1975, *32,* 439–443.

Brown, G. W., & Harris, T. *Social origins of depression.* London: Tavistock, 1978.

Buck, R. *The communication of emotion.* New York: Guilford Press, 1984.

Buchsbaum, M. S., Ingvar, D. H., Kessler, R., Waters, R. N., Cappeletti, J., van Konner, D. P., King, A. C., Johnsch, J. L., Manning, R. G., Flynn, R. W., Mann, L. S., Bummey, W. E., Jr., & Sokoloff, L. Cerebral glucography with position tomography: Use in normal subjects and in patients with schizophrenia. *Archives of General Psychiatry,* 1982, *39,* 251–259.

Buie, J. "Me" decades generate depression. *The APA Monitor,* Oct. 1988, p. 18.

Bouthol, G. *La Guerre.* Paris: Presses Universitaire, 1969.

Cannon, W. B. Vodoo death. *American Anthropologist.* 1949, 44(2).

Cannon, W. B. The James-Lange theory of emotions: A critical examination and an alternative theory. *American Journal of Psychology,* 1927, *39,* 106–124.

Connors K., *et al.* Children of parents with affective disorders. *Journal of Child Psychiatry,* 1979, *18,* 600–607.

Cooper, A. Will neurobiology influence psychoanalysis? *American Journal of Psychiatry,* 1985, *142,* 1395–1402.

Cotman, C. W. (Ed.). *Synaptic plasticity.* New York: Guilford Press, 1987.

Von Cranach, M., Koppa, K., Lepanis, W., & Ploog, P. (Eds.). *Human ethology, claims and limits of a new discipline.* Cambridge, UK: Cambridge University Press, 1979.

Davidson, J. M., & Davidson, R. J. (Eds.). *The psychobiology of consciousness.* New York: Plenum Press, 1980.

de Saint Exupéry, A. *The little prince.* (K. Woods, trans.). New York: Harcourt, Brace and World, 1943.

Dewey, J. *Experience and nature.* New York: Dover Books, 1958.

Dewey, J. *Human nature and conduct.* New York: Holt, 1922.

DiMascio, A., & Shader, R. (Eds.). *Clinical handbook of psychopharmacology.* New York: Science House, 1970.

Durkheim, E. *Le Suicide.* Paris: Libraire Felix Alcan, 1897.

Ehrhartd, A. A. The psychobiology of gender. In A. Rossi (Ed.), *Gender and the life course.* New York: Aldine, 1985.

Eisdorfer, C., Cohen, D., Kleinman, A., & Maxim, P. *Models for Clinical Psychopathology.* New York: Spectrum, 1981.

Eitinger, L. A follow-up study of Norwegian concentration camp survivors, mortality and morbidity. *The Israel Annals of Psychiatry and Related Disciplines,* 1973, *11*(3).

Ernst, E., & Goodison, L. *In our own hands.* London: Women's Press, 1981.

Fairbairn, W. R. D. *Psychoanalytic studies of personality.* London: Tavistock, 1952.

Favazza, A. R. Little murders. *The Sciences,* March 1989, 5–7.

Feather, N. T., & Barber, J. G. Depressive reactions, and unemployment. *Journal of Abnormal Psychology,* 1983, *92*, 185–195.

Flach, F. (Ed.). Psychobiology and psychopharmacology. New York: Norton, 1988.

Freedman, D. X. (Ed.). *Biology and the major psychoses.* New York: Raven Press, 1975.

Freud, S. *An outline of psychoanalysis.* (J. Strachey, Ed. and trans.) New York: Norton, 1949.

Fry, W. H., & Langeth, M. *Crying; the mystery of tears.* New York: Winston Press, 1985.

Fromm, E. *The forgotten language.* New York: Grove Press, 1951.

Fromm, E. Die psychoanalytische Characterologie und ihre Bedeutung fur die Sozialpsychologie. *Zeitschrift fur Sozialforschung,* 1932, *3*, 253–277.

Fromm-Reichman, F. An intensive study of twelve cases of manic depressive psychosis. In *Psychoanalysis and psychotherapy:*

selected papers. Chicago, IL: University of Chicago Press, 1959.

Gardner, R. Mechanisms in manic depressive disorders: An evolutionary model. *Archives of General Psychiatry,* 1982, *39,* 1327–1333.

Gaylin, W. *Caring.* New York: Knopf, 1976.

Gedo, J., & Goldberg, A. *Models of the mind.* Chicago, IL: University of Chicago Press, 1973.

Gold, M. S. *The good news about depression.* New York: Villard Books, 1987.

Goleman, D. Opoids and denial: Two mechanisms for bypassing pain. *Advances,* 1985, *2*(2).

Goldhammer, P. Psychotherapy and pharmacotherapy: The challenge of integration. *Canadian Journal of Psychiatry,* 1983, *28,* 173–177.

Gray, J. A. *The neuropsychology of anxiety: An enquiry into functions of the septo-hippocampal system.* New York: Oxford University Press, 1982.

Greenacre, P. *Affective disorders.* New York: International Universities Press, 1953.

Greenfield, N. S., & Lewis, W. C. *Psychoanalysis and current biological thought.* Madison, WI: University of Wisconsin Press, 1965.

Harlow, H. S. The nature of love. *American Psychologist,* 1958, *13,* 673–685.

Harlow, H. F. *Learning to love.* San Francisco, CA: Albion Press, 1971.

Haim, I., & Usdin, E. *Animal models in psychiatry and neurology.* Oxford, UK: Pergamon Press, 1977.

Haracz, J. Neural plasticity and inclusion of biology in psychoanalytic metatheory. *Psychoanalysis and Contemporary Thought,* 1984, *7*(4), 469–490.

Hays, P. Etiological factors in manic-depressive psychoses. *Archives of General Psychiatry,* 1976, *33,* 1187–1188.

Heilman, K. M., & Satz, P. (Eds.). *Neuropsychology of human emotions.* New York: Guilford Press, 1983.

Helfer, R. A., & Kempe, H. C. (Eds.). *The battered child*. Chicago, IL: University of Chicago Press, 1968.

Hersne, M., Bellak, A. S., & Himmelhoch, J. M. Treatment of unipolar depression with social skills training. *Behavior Modification*, 1980, *4*, 549–556.

Himmelhoch, J. M. Mixed states, manic depressive illness, and the nature of mood. *Psychiatric Clinics of North America*, 1979, *2*, 449–459.

Hooper, J., & Teresi, D. *The three-pound universe*. New York: Dell Publishing, 1986.

Izard, C. E. A. (Ed.). *Emotions in personality and psychopathology*. New York: Plenum Press, 1979.

Jackson, S. W. *Melancholia and depression*. New Haven: Yale University Press, 1986.

Jacobson, E. *Depression*. New York: International Universities Press, 1971.

Jacobson, E. *The self and the object world*. New York: International Universities Press, 1973.

Jahoda, M. The impact of unemployment in the 1930's and the 1970's. *Bulletin of British Psychological Sociology*, 1979, *32*, 309–314.

James, W. *Principles of psychology*. New York: Holt, 1890.

John, E. R., Prichep, L. S., Friedman, J., & Easton, P. Neurometrics: Computer-assisted differential diagnosis of brain dysfunctions. *Science*, 1988, *239*, 162–169.

Janowsky, D., Leff, M., & Epstein, R. Playing the manic game. *Archives of General Psychiatry*, 1970, *22*, 252–265.

Johnson, G. Memory, learning, how it works. *The New York Times Magazine*, Aug. 9, 1987.

Kandel, E. R. Psychotherapy and the single synapse: The impact of psychiatric thought on neurobiological research. *New England Journal of Medicine*, 1979, *301*, 1028–1037.

Kandel, E. R. Genes, nerve cells and the remembrance of things past. *Journal of Neuropsychiatry*, 1989, *2*, 103–125.

Katz, R. J. Animal models and human depressive disorders. *Biobehavioral Review*, 1981, *5*, 231–246.

Kesey, K. *One flew over the cuckoo's nest*. New York: Viking Press, 1962.

Khan, M. M. R. *The privacy of the self*. New York: International Universities Press, 1974.

Khan, M. M. R. *Alienation in perversions*. New York: International Universities Press, 1979.

Klein, D. F. Endogenomorphic depression: A conceptual and terminological revision. *Archives of General Psychiatry*, 1974, *31*, 447–454.

Klein, D. F., Fencil-Morse, E., & Seligman, M. E. P. Learned helplessness, depression and attribution of failure. *Journal of Personality and Social Psychology*, 1976, *33*, 508–516.

Klein, D. F., Gittelman, R., Quitkin, F., & Rifkin, A. *Diagnosis and drug treatment of psychiatric disorders: Adults and children* (2nd ed.). Baltimore, MD: Williams and Wilkins, 1980.

Klein, M. A contribution to the psychogenesis of manic-depressive states. In *Contributions to psychoanalysis*. London: Hogarth Press, 1948.

Kingsbury, S. J. Cognitive differences between clinical psychologists and psychiatrists. *American Psychologist*, 1988, *42*(2), 152–156.

Klerman, G. L., Prusoff, B. A., *et al.* Depressed outpatients one year after treatment with drugs and/or interpersonal psychiatry (I.P.T.). *Archives of General Psychiatry*, 1981, *38*, 51–55.

Klerman, G. L., Weissman, M., Ronnsaville, B. J., & Chevron, E. S. *Interpersonal psychotherapy of depression*. New York: Basic Books, 1984.

Klerman, G. L., & Myers, J. K. Affective disorders in a United States community: The use of research diagnostic criteria in an epidemiological survey. *Archives of General Psychiatry*, 1978, *35*, 1304–1311.

Kline, N. S. *From sad to glad*. New York: Ballantine Books, 1974.

Kluckhohn, C. *Culture and behavior*. Glencoe, IL: Free Press, 1962.

Kobler, A. L., & Stotland, E. *The end of hope*. Glencoe, IL: Free Press, 1964.

Kohut, H. *The analysis of the self*. New York: International Universities Press, 1971.

Kohut, H. *The restoration of the self*. New York: International Universities Press, 1977.

Konner, M. *The tangled wing: Biological constraints on the human spirit*. New York: Holt, Rinehart & Winston, 1982.

Konner, M. *Becoming a doctor*. New York: Viking Press, 1987.

Kovacs, M. Efficacy of cognitive and behavior therapies for depression. *American Journal of Psychiatry*, 1980; *137*, 1495–1501.

Krauthammer, C., & Klerman, G. L. The epidemiology of mania. In Shopsin, B. (Ed.). *Manic illness*. New York: Raven Press, 1979.

Lash, C. *The culture of narcissism*. New York: Norton, 1979.

Leak, G. K., & Christopher, S. B. Freudian psychoanalysis and sociobiology: A synthesis. *American Psychologist*, 1982, *37*, 313–332.

Lear, F. Color me blue. *Lears*, 1989, 2 (2), April.

Levi, P. *The drowned and the saved*. New York: Summit Books, 1988.

Lewis, M., & Rosenblum, L. A. *The development of affect*. New York: Plenum Press, 1978.

Lewontin, R. C., Rose, S., & Kamin, L. J. *Not in our genes*. New York: Pantheon Books, 1984.

Lichtenberg, J. D. *Psychoanalysis and infant research*. Hillsdale, NJ: The Analytic Press, 1983.

Lickey, M. E., & Gordon, B. *Drugs for mental illness*. New York: W. H. Freeman, 1983.

Lloyd, C. Life events and depressive disorders reviewed, I. Events as predisposing factors. *Archives of General Psychiatry*, 1980a, *37*, 529–535.

Lloyd, C. Life events and depressive disorders reviewed, II. Events as predisposing factors. *Archives of General Psychiatry*, 1980b, *37*, 541–548.

Lin, N., Dean, A., & Ensel, W. (Eds.). *Social support, life events, and depression*. New York: Academic Press, 1986.

Lipsitt, L. P. (Ed.). *Developmental psychobiology.* New York: Erlbaum, 1976.

Loeb, F., & Loeb, L. R. Psychoanalytic observations on the effect of lithium on manic attacks. *Journal of the American Psychoanalytic Association,* 1988, 35(4), 877–902.

Lopata Znaniecki, H. *Widowhood in an American city.* Morristown, NJ: General Learning Press, 1973.

Lorenz, K. *King Salomon's ring: New light on animal's ways.* New York: Thomas Y. Crowell, 1952.

Luchterhand, E. Survival in concentration camps: An individual or group phenomenon. In Rosenberg, I. G. and Howton, F. W. (Eds.), *Mass society in crisis: Social problems and social pathology.* New York: Macmillan, 1964.

Mahler, M. S. *On human symbiosis and the vicissitudes of individuation.* New York: International Universities Press, 1968.

Mahler, M. S., Pine, F., & Berman, A. *The psychological birth of the human infant.* New York: Basic Books, 1975.

Marsella, A. J., Hirshfield, R. M. A., & Katz, M. M. (Eds.). *The measurement of depression.* New York: Guilford Press, 1987.

McLean, P. D. Psychosomatic medicine and the visceral brain: Recent developments bearing on Papez' theory of emotion. *Psychosomatic Medicine,* 1949, 11, 338–353.

McLean, P. D., & Hakstian, L. Clinical depression; Comparative efficacy of outpatient treatments. *Journal of Consulting Clinical Psychology,* 1979, 47, 818–836.

Mead, G. H. *Mind, self and society.* Chicago, IL: University of Chicago Press, 1934.

Merton, R. K. *Social theory and social structure.* Glencoe, IL: Free Press, 1957.

Miller, S. *The shame experience.* Hillsdale, NJ: The Analytic Press, 1985.

Miller, T. W. (Ed.). *Stressful life events.* Madison, CT: International Universities Press, 1989.

Miller, J. G. *Living systems.* New York: McGraw Hill, 1978.

Murdock, G. P. *Ethnographic atlas.* Pittsburgh, PA: University of Pittsburgh Press, 1967.

Ornstein, R., & Thompson, R. F. *The amazing brain*. Boston, MA: Houghton Mifflin, 1984.

Parens, H., & Saul, L. J. *Dependence in man: A psychoanalytic study*. New York: International Universities Press, 1971.

Paykel, E. S. (Ed.). *Handbook of affective disorders*. New York: Guilford Press, 1982.

Pert, C. D. The wisdom of the receptors: Neuropeptides, the emotions and body mind. *Advances*, 1986, *3*(3), 8–16.

Pine, F. The four psychologies of psychoanalysis and their place in clinical work. *Journal of the American Psychoanalytic Association*, 1988, *36*(3), 571–596.

Pine, F. *Developmental theory and clinical process*. New Haven, CT: Yale University Press, 1985.

Plutchik, R., & Kellerman, H. (Eds.). *Emotion: theory, research, and experience*. New York: Academic Press, 1980.

Pisar, S. *Of blood and hope*. New York: Macmillan, 1979.

Post, R. M. Clinical implications of a cocaine-kindling model of psychosis. In H. L. Klawans (Ed.), *Clinical neuropharmacology* (Vol. 2). New York: Raven Press, 1977.

Price, J. The dominance hierarchy and the evolution of mental illness. *Lancet*, 1967, *2*, 243–246.

Des Pres, T. *The survivor: An anatomy of life in the death camps*. New York: Oxford University Press, 1976.

Parisi, T. Why Freud failed; Some implications for neurophysiology and sociobiology. *American Psychologist*, 1987, *42*(3), 235–245.

Papez, J. W. A proposed mechanism of emotion. *Archives of Neurological Psychiatry*, 1937, *38*, 725–743.

Piaget, J. *The child and reality*. New York: Penguin Books, 1976.

Piaget, J., & Inhelder, B. *The psychology of the child*. New York: Basic Books, 1966.

Nicholi, A. M., Jr. (Ed.). *The Harvard guide to modern psychiatry*. Cambridge MA: Harvard University Press, 1978.

Normand, W. C., & Bluestone, H. The use of pharmacotherapy in psychoanalytic treatment. *Contemporary Psychoanalysis*, 1986, *22*(2), 218–234.

Radke-Yarrow, M. *Risk and protective factors in the development of psychopathology.* Cambridge, UK: Cambridge University Press, 1989.

Reiser, M. F. *Mind, brain, body.* New York: Basic Books, 1984.

Rieber, R. W. (Ed.). *Body and mind, past, present, and future.* New York: Academic Press, 1980.

Rogawski, A. S. A systems theoretical approach to the understanding of emotions. *Journal of the American Academy of Psychoanalysis,* 1987, *15,*(2), 133–151.

Rosenzweig, E. B., & Diamond, M. C. Brain changes in response to experience. *Scientific American,* 1972, *226,* 22–29.

Rosenzweig, N., & Griscorn, H. (Eds.). *Psycho-pharmacology and psychotherapy: Synthesis or antithesis?* New York: Human Sciences Press, 1987.

Rossi, A. (Ed.). *Gender and the life course.* New York: Aldine, 1985.

Rossi, E. L. *The psychobiology of mind-body healing.* New York: Norton, 1986.

Rossi, E. L. From mind to molecule: State dependent learning and behavior theory of mind body healing. *Advances,* 1987, *4*(2), 46–60.

Rossi, E. L., & Cheek, D. B. *Mind-body therapy.* New York: Norton, 1988.

Rushdie, S. *Shame.* New York: Knopf, 1983.

Sameroff, A. J., & Emde, R. (Eds.). *Relationship disturbances in early childhood.* New York: Basic Books, 1989.

Sander, L. W. Adaptative relationships in early mother child interaction. *Journal of the American Academy of Child Psychiatry,* 1964, *3,* 231–264.

Sapolski, R. M. Lessons of the Serengeti. *Science,* 1988, *126,* 38–42.

Schachter, S., & Singer, J. E. Cognitive, social and physiological determinants of emotional states. *Psychological Review,* 1962, *69,* 379–399.

Schad, S. P. *Empirical social research in Weimar Germany.* The Hague: Mouton Co., 1972.

Schad-Somers, S. P. *Sadomasochism: Etiology and treatment*. New York: Human Sciences Press, 1982.

Schmale, A. H., & Engel, G. L. The role of conservation-withdrawal in depressive reactions. In E. J. Anthony and T. Benedek (Eds.), *Depression and human existence*. Boston, MA: Little, Brown, 1975.

Searles, H. *Collected papers on schizophrenia and related subjects*. New York: International Universities Press, 1965.

Seligman, M. E. P., & Hager, J. L. Biological boundaries of learning. New York: Appleton Century Crofts, 1972.

Senay, E. C. General systems theory and depression. *American Association for the Advancement of Science*, 1973, 242–273.

Singer, J. L. *Imagery and daydreams in psychotherapy and behavior modification*. New York: Academic Press, 1974.

Simons, R. C. Psychoanalytic contributions to psychiatric nosology; Forms of masochistic behavior. *Journal of the American Psychoanalytic Association*, 1987, 35(3), 583–608.

Solomon, G. F. The emerging field of psychoimmunology with a special note on AIDS. *Advances*, 1985, 2(1).

Sonnier, B. J. Quantitative analysis of the development of cortical stellate cells: Differences related to rearing environments of monkeys. (M. Arctoides). Unpublished doctoral dissertation. Riverside, CA: University of California, 1981.

Speigel, R., & Aebi, H-J. *Psychopharmacology: An introduction*. New York: Wiley, 1984.

Spiegelstein, M. G., & Levy, A. *Behavioral models and the analysis of Drug action*. Amsterdam, The Netherlands: Elsevier, 1982.

Spitz, R. A. *The genetic field theory of ego formation*. New York: International University Press, 1959.

Spitz, R. A. *The first year of life*. New York: International Universities Press, 1965.

Stern, D. N. *The interpersonal world of the infant*. New York: Basic Books, 1985.

Stoddard, J. B., & Henry, J. P. Affectional bonding and the impact of bereavement, *Advances*, 1985, 2(2), 19–28.

Stoller, R. J. *Perversion*. New York: Dell, 1975.

Stoller, R. J. *Sex and Gender* (Vol. 2). New York: Jason Aronson, 1968.

Stone, M. H. Mania: A guide for the perplexed. *Psychiatry and Social Science Review,* 1971, *5,* 14–18.

Stone, M. H. Toward early detection of manic depressive illness in psychoanalytic patients. *American Journal of Psychotherapy,* 1978, *32,* 427–439.

Stone, M. H. *The borderline syndromes.* New York: McGraw-Hill, 1980.

Stolorow, R. D., & Lachmann, F. M. *Psychoanalysis of developmental arrests.* New York: International Universities Press, 1980.

Styron, W. Why Primo Levi need not have died. Op. Ed. *The New York Times,* Dec. 19, 1988.

Sumners, M. *The Malleus Malifecarum.* London: The Folio Society, 1968.

Thompson, J. G. *The psychobiology of emotions.* New York: Plenum Press, 1988.

Tiger, L. *Optimism: The biology of hope.* New York: Simon & Schuster, 1979.

Tsen, Wen-Shin, & Mc Dermott, J. F. *Culture, mind and therapy.* New York: Bruner Mazel, 1981.

Val, E. R., Gavira, F. M., & Flaherty, J. A. *Affective disorders: Psychopathology and treatment.* Chicago, IL: Yearbook Medical Publishers, 1932.

Willner, P. *Depression, a psychobiological synthesis.* New York: Wiley Interscience, 1985.

Wender, P. H., & Klein, D. F. *Mind, mood and medicine.* New York: New American Library, 1981.

Weiss, J. M. Psychological factors in stress and disease. *Scientific American,* 1972, *226,* 104–113.

Weiss, J. M., Baily, W. H., Goodman, P. A., Hoffman, L. J. Ambrose, M. J., Salman, S., & Charry, J. M. A model for the neurochemical study of depression. In M. Y. Spiegelstein & A. Levy (Eds.), *Behavioral model and the analysis of drug action.* Amsterdam, The Netherlands: Elsevier, 1982.

Weisskopf, V. The origin of the universe. *New York Review of Books* (Vol. XXXVI), 1989, 2, 10–14.

Weissman, M., *et al.* Symptom patterns in primary and secondary depression; A comparison of primary depressives with depressed opiate addicts, alcoholics and schizophrenics. *Archives General Psychiatry*, 1977, 34, 854–862.

Whybrow, P. C., Akiskal, H. S., & McKinney, Jr., W. T. *Mood disorders.* New York: Plenum Press, 1984.

Winnicott, D. W. Transitional objects and transitional phenomena. *International Journal of Psychoanalysis*, 1953, 34, 89–97.

Winnicott, D. W. *The maturational processes and the facilitating environment.* New York: International Universities Press, 1965.

Witenberg, E. G. (Ed.) *Interpersonal psychoanalysis.* New York: Gardner Press, 1978.

Wolpert, E. A. *Manic depressive illness as an actual neurosis.* New York: International Universities Press, 1977.

Wulsin, L., Bachop, M., & Hoffman, D. Group therapy in manic depressive illness. *American Journal of Psychotherapy* (Vol. XLII), 1988, 2, 263–271.

Yapko, M. D. *When living hurts.* New York: Bruner Mazel, 1988.

Young, P. T. *Emotion in man and animal: Its nature and dynamic basis.* Huntington, NY: Robert E. Krieger, 1973.

Zeiss, A. M., Levinson, P. M., & Munoz, R. F. Nonspecific improvement effects in depression using interpersonal skills training, pleasant activity schedules, or cognitive training. *Journal of Consulting Clinical Psychology*, 1979, 45, 543–551.

Znaiecky-Lopata, H. *Widowhood in an American city.* Cambridge, MA: Schenckman, 1973.

Zohar, D. *The quantum self.* New York: William Morrow and Co., 1990.

Index